For Fred Silva,

With fond wishes.

Errol

Come & see us some
time !

D0858250

From Rags to Riches

FROM RAGS TO RICHES

The Phenomenal Rise of the University of Texas
Southwestern Medical Center at Dallas

Errol C. Friedberg

CAROLINA ACADEMIC PRESS
Durham, North Carolina

Copyright © 2007 Errol C. Friedberg
All Rights Reserved.

Library of Congress Cataloging-in-Publication Data

Friedberg, Errol C.
From rags to riches : the phenomenal rise of the University of
Texas Southwestern Medical Center at Dallas / by Errol C. Friedberg.
    p. ; cm.
Includes bibliographical references and index.
ISBN-13: 978-1-59460-397-6 (alk. paper)
ISBN-10: 1-59460-397-9 (alk. paper)
  1. University of Texas Southwestern Medical Center at Dallas--
History. 2. Medical colleges--Texas--Dallas--History. I. Title.
    [DNLM: 1. University of Texas Southwestern Medical Center at
Dallas. 2. Schools, Medical--history--Texas. 3. Biomedical
Research--history--Texas. 4. Faculty, Medical--history--Texas.
W 19 F911f 2007]

R747.U6853F75 2007
610.71'1097642812--dc22   2007001308

Carolina Academic Press
700 Kent Street
Durham, NC 27701
Telephone (919) 489-7486
Fax (919) 493-5668
www.cap-press.com

Printed in the United States of America

To Donald W. Seldin

A redoubtable University of Texas Southwestern pioneer

CONTENTS

Preface
xi

Timeline
xiii

CHAPTER 1
A Fourth Nobel Prize
3

CHAPTER 2
Early Medical Education and Research in the United States
9

CHAPTER 3
The Birth of a Medical School in Dallas
17

CHAPTER 4
The University of Texas Southwestern Medical School
41

CHAPTER 5
The Early Seldin Years
49

CHAPTER 6
Charles Cameron Sprague—A Milk-Drinking Texas Boy
71

CHAPTER 7

The First Nobel Laureates

99

CHAPTER 8

Expanding in Difficult Times—The Wildenthal Years

125

CHAPTER 9

Portraits of Some Prominent Dallas Philanthropists

137

CHAPTER 10

The North Campus Development: A Showpiece for the Future

157

CHAPTER 11

Epilogue

165

APPENDIX

Distinguished UT Southwestern Faculty Members

169

Notes

171

Index

175

Why not a great medical center in Dallas?

Edward H. Cary, *Dean, University of Dallas Medical Department*

The medical school, at the outset of the 1950s had almost no financial resources whatsoever, and the facilities were poor. It was an opportunity as well as a problem. Fortunately, we had resources of a kind which should be remembered; we had students; we had housestaff; and we had student fellows. They would be, ultimately, the faculty of the future.

Donald W. Seldin, *Chairman Emeritus, Department of Internal Medicine, Southwestern Medical School of the University of Texas*

I don't believe that the work that Joe and I have done could have been done at any other institution, because no other institution has the combination of assets and people that have made it possible.

Michael S. Brown, *Nobel Laureate, Department of Molecular Genetics, University of Texas Southwestern Medical School*

The goal of UT Southwestern is to identify, recruit, and retain the top educators, physicians, and researchers in the world, provide them with an environment that will enable them to flourish; and encourage them to think boldly and build programs that will be the best of their kind anywhere. That philosophy, coupled with the support of community philanthropists and Texas political leaders has created an institution that is the envy of our peers around the world.

Kern Wildenthal, *President, University of Texas Southwestern Medical Center at Dallas*

Preface

After spending close to two decades on the faculty at Stanford University Medical School, my decision to move to a considerably less well-known academic institution located in a state infamous, for, among other things, its torrid summers, was, to say the least, problematical. Forgetting for the moment my concurrence with all that I have heard about summers in Texas, being a faculty member at the University of Texas Southwestern (UT Southwestern) Medical Center has without question been the most satisfying and rewarding experience of my academic career.

I came quickly to understand that an intense pride and commitment permeates the halls of this extraordinary academic medical school, so much so that I was prompted to scrutinize and ultimately to document UT Southwestern's astonishing ascendancy from arguably the most humble beginnings of any medical school in the country—certainly in the modern era. In so doing I have labored to avoid the format of dry historical documentation, striving instead to offer what I hope is a palpable flavor of some of the many personalities who contributed so profoundly to UT Southwestern's rise from also-ran to academic front-runner. Thus, I make no claims here for historical completeness. Instead, *From Rags to Riches* is for the most part a story about people. While practical reasons dictated that my recounting necessarily focus on a restricted set of prominent personalities, UT Southwestern owes its present reputation for academic excellence both to a much larger cadre of distinguished faculty and staff and to a loyal and dedicated group of Dallas citizens. I urge readers to examine the timeline provided for some notable events that transpired during the past century and to peruse previous historical offerings, notably *The University of Texas Southwestern Medical School: Medical Education in Dallas, 1900–1975* by former UT Southwestern faculty member John Chapman, and a comprehensive pictorial reminiscence by George Race called *UT Southwestern—Commemorating the First Half Century.*

My reportage may be accused of bias in favor of the basic science community at this institution. I plead guilty. But while it is an incontrovertible fact that UT Southwestern's most spectacular academic successes have (to date) indeed been in the basic science arena, it should be noted that three of its four Nobel laureates are trained physicians, and that two of them pursued formal residency and fellowship training in Internal Medicine. Furthermore, as this book reveals, UT Southwestern's earliest claims to fame were in fact in the area of academic medicine, not the basic sciences per se. This caveat aside, UT Southwestern also enjoys an important position in the pantheon of clinical medicine, and future developments in this area, some of which have been initiated at the time of this writing, will certainly enhance this position.

In documenting this medical school's history, I relied heavily on personal interviews. I am grateful to Mike Brown, Burton Combes, Johann Deisenhofer, Ron Estabrook, John Fordtran, Al Gilman, Joe Goldstein, Mary McDermott Cook, Steve McKnight, Peter O'Donnell, Ross Perot, Don Seldin, Jonathan Uhr, Kern Wildenthal, and Jean Wilson for their unstinting time and interest. I also thank my wife Rhonda for her constant cheerleading and her indispensable evaluation of innumerable drafts, and Angela Ceplis, Meredith Thomas, and Wendy Deaner for their secretarial and logistical help.

I owe heart-felt thanks to Neil Patterson, who, convinced of the imperative to publish this book, orchestrated critical contacts with Carolina Academic Press. Thanks also to Keith Sipe and his able staff (in particular Tim Colton) at Carolina Academic Press for their outstanding assistance, to Penny Austen for her expert editing, to Dr. Keith Wharton and Nicole Kosarek for their reading and proofing of the manuscript, to Wes Norred, Cyndi Bassel, Nancy Potter, Bill Maina, David Gresham, and Karen Vieth at UT Southwestern for their assistance in procuring photographs and to Mark Smith for reproducing them for publication. Bill Maina and Laurie Thompson at the UT Southwestern library provided crucial help. Finally, I thank Dr. Kern Wildenthal, president of UT Southwestern Medical Center at Dallas for his enthusiastic support, his commitment to conscientiously offering comments and suggestions on numerous drafts, and his invaluable help in promoting the publication of this work.

Errol C. Friedberg, MD
September 2006

TIMELINE

1900   The University of Dallas Medical Department is established as the first medical school in Dallas, with founder **Charles M. Rosser** as dean. Hospital affiliation is with the Good Samaritan Hospital. Within a few months, a splinter group establishes the rival Dallas Medical College.

1901   **Edward H. Cary** becomes Dean of the University of Dallas Medical Department.

1903   The University of Dallas Medical Department becomes Baylor University Medical College, enjoying formal affiliation with Baylor University in Waco, Texas. **Edward H. Cary** is the first dean. Hospital affiliation is with Baylor University Hospital, formerly Texas Baptist Memorial Sanitarium.

1910   **Abraham Flexner** publishes *Medical Education in the United States and Canada*, a report on the state of American and Canadian medical schools. The report has far-reaching consequences for many medical schools.

1913   **Parkland Hospital**, opened in 1894, becomes affiliated with Baylor University Medical College.

1939   The **Southwestern Medical Foundation** is founded in Dallas.

1943   Baylor Medical College moves to Houston and **Southwestern Medical College** is established in Dallas by the Southwestern Medical Foundation. The school is located in army barracks on Oak Lawn Avenue and is the 68th medical school in the U.S.

           Donald Slaughter is appointed the first Dean of **Southwestern Medical College.**

1943/44 The school's annual budget is approximately $200,000.

1944   **Tinsley R. Harrison** is appointed Chairman of the Department of Internal Medicine and Dean of the Medical School, and begins writing *Principles of Internal Medicine.*

1945   **S. Edward Sulkin** is appointed Chairman of the Department of Microbiology.

1946   **William Lee Hart** is appointed Dean of the medical school.

      Carl A. Moyer is appointed Professor of Experimental Surgery in the Department of Surgery.

      Arthur Grollman is appointed Chairman of the Departments of Physiology and Pharmacology.

1949   Southwestern Medical College becomes part of the University of Texas System and changes its name to **Southwestern Medical School of the University of Texas.** The school's annual budget is about $500,000.

1950   **Tinsley R. Harrison** leaves Southwestern Medical College.

      Carl A. Moyer is appointed Dean of Southwestern Medical College.

1951   **Donald W. Seldin** arrives in Dallas as a junior faculty member in the Department of Internal Medicine under Chairman **Charles Burnett.** Burnett departs less than a year later, leaving the Department of Internal Medicine with but two full-time faculty members.

1952   **James Aagaard** is appointed Dean of Southwestern Medical School.

      Donald W. Seldin is appointed Acting Chairman of the Department of Internal Medicine at Southwestern Medical School and the following year is named as permanent chairman.

1954   **James A. Gill** succeeds James Aagaard as Dean of the Medical School.

      A new **Parkland Hospital** opens on Harry Hines Boulevard.

1955   The first new building on the site presently occupied by the medical center is opened adjacent to the new Parkland Hospital and is named the **Edward H. Cary Building for Basic Sciences.**

1958   A second new building, the **Karl Hoblitzelle Building for Clinical Sciences,** opens its doors. The clinical departments move from the old shacks on Oak Lawn Avenue to the present location on Harry Hines Boulevard.

1962   Joseph L. Goldstein, future Nobel laureate, enters medical school at Southwestern.

1965–75   The entering medical school class is expanded from 100 to 200 students.

            The **Dan Danciger Research Building** opens.

1967   **Charles C. Sprague** is appointed Dean of the Medical School. The school's annual budget is now approximately $10 million.

            The senior class attains top place in the country on Part II of the National Board Examinations.

1968   **Children's Medical Center** moves to the UT Southwestern campus.

1970–80   The campus is expanded by ~500,000 nsf with the addition of the **Philip R. Jonsson Basic Science Research Building,** the **Eugene McDermott Academic Administration Building,** the **Tom and Lula Gooch Auditorium,** the **Eugene McDermott Plaza and Lecture Rooms,** the **Cecil H. and Ida Green Science Building,** the **Fred F. Florence Bioinformation Center,** and the **Harry S. Moss Clinical Science Building.**

            Ronald W. Estabrook is appointed Chairman of the Department of Biochemistry.

1971   **Rupert E. Billingham,** Fellow of the Royal Society of London, is appointed Chairman of the Department of Cell Biology.

            Michael S. Brown, future Nobel laureate, becomes a post-doctoral fellow in the Department of Internal Medicine and a year later joins the faculty.

1972   The Medical Center, now comprising a medical school, a graduate school and a School of Allied Health Sciences, is renamed the **University of Texas Health Sciences Center at Dallas.**

            Charles Cameron Sprague becomes the center's first president.

1973   **Fred Bonte** becomes Dean of the Medical School.

            Jonathan W. Uhr is appointed Chairman of the Department of Microbiology.

            Joseph L. Goldstein joins the faculty of the Department of Internal Medicine.

1979   **Ronald W. Estabrook** is elected to the U.S. National Academy of Sciences.

1980   Michael S. Brown and Joseph L. Goldstein are elected to the U.S. National Academy of Sciences.

Kern Wildenthal succeeds Fred Bonte as Dean of the Medical School.

1980–90   Another 300,000 nsf of academic space is added to the medical center with the completion of the Cecil H. and Ida Green Science Building and the Charles Cameron Sprague Clinical Science Building.

1981   Alfred G. Gilman is appointed Chairman of the Department of Pharmacology.

1983   Jean D. Wilson, of the Department of Internal Medicine, is elected to the U.S. National Academy of Sciences.

1984   Jonathan W. Uhr is elected to the U.S. National Academy of Sciences.

The Aston Ambulatory Center opens its doors.

1985   Michael S. Brown and Joseph L. Goldstein are awarded the Nobel Prize in Physiology or Medicine.

Alfred G. Gilman is elected to the U.S. National Academy of Sciences.

The medical school is designated a member of the Howard Hughes Medical Institute.

1986   Kern Wildenthal is appointed the second President of the UT Southwestern Medical Center at Dallas.

William B. Neaves becomes Dean of the Medical School.

Roger H. Unger, of the Department of Internal Medicine, is elected to the U.S. National Academy of Sciences.

1987   The Medical Center once again changes its name, this time becoming The University of Texas Southwestern Medical Center at Dallas, the name it presently holds.

The UT Southwestern Medical Center acquires land from the John D. and Catherine T. MacArthur Foundation and planning begins for the future North Campus.

1988   Johann Deisenhofer, of the Department of Biochemistry, is awarded the Nobel Prize in Chemistry.

1989   Zale Lipshy University Hospital opens its doors.

1990–2000   New facilities totaling over 600,000 nsf, comprising the **Simmons, Hamon** and **Seay Biomedical Research Buildings**, are completed on the North Campus.

1993   **David L. Garbers,** in the Department of Pharmacology, is elected to the U.S. National Academy of Sciences.

The first **North Campus** building opens.

1994   **Alfred G. Gilman** is awarded the Nobel Prize in Physiology or Medicine.

Ellen Vitetta, in the Department of Microbiology, is elected to the U.S. National Academy of Sciences.

1995   **Steven L. McKnight,** a member of the U.S. National Academy of Sciences, is appointed Chairman of the Department of Biochemistry.

1999   **Robert J. Alpern** is appointed Dean of the Medical School.

2000   **Eric N. Olson,** Chairman of the Department of Molecular Biology, is elected to the U.S. National Academy of Sciences.

St. Paul Medical Center is acquired by UT Southwestern Medical Center and is leased to Zale Lipshy University Hospital, which renames it **St. Paul University Hospital at Southwestern Medical Center.**

2000–2006   Three additional buildings totaling ~500,000 nsf, the **Moncrief Radiation Oncology Building,** the **Bill and Rita Clements Advanced Medical Imaging Building** and the 14-story **Biomedical Research Tower,** are completed on the North Campus.

2002   **Thomas C. Sudhof,** of the Neurosciences Center, is elected to the U.S. National Academy of Sciences.

2003   **Masashi Yanagisawa,** of the Department of Molecular Genetics, is elected to the U.S. National Academy of Sciences.

2004   **Xiaodong Wang,** of the Department of Biochemistry, is elected to the U.S. National Academy of Sciences.

Alfred G. Gilman is appointed Dean of the Medical School.

2005   UT Southwestern Medical Center acquires **Zale Lipshy University Hospital** and **St. Paul University Hospital,** merges them as **UT Southwestern University Hospitals,** and assumes full responsibility for their operations and finances.

2006   **Alfred G. Gilman** is appointed Provost of the University and Executive Vice-President for Academic Affairs.

David W. Russell of the Department of Molecular Genetics and **Melanie Cobb** of the Department of Pharmacology are elected to the U.S. National Academy of Sciences.

Xiaodong Wang of the Department of Biochemistry wins the one million-dollar Shaw Prize in Life Science and Medicine.

The operating budget is over $1.2 billion.

FROM RAGS TO RICHES

CHAPTER 1

A FOURTH NOBEL PRIZE

News that the UT Southwestern Medical Center was to have a fourth Nobel laureate in its faculty arrived in the traditional manner. In the wee hours of October 10, 1994, Alfred Goodman (Al) Gilman was awakened by a phone call from Stockholm. "When the phone rang at 5:15 in the morning I knew what it was about," he related. "Still, it was a shock."[1] Later that day, the Nobel Foundation announced that the award would be given to Gilman and Martin Rodbell (from the National Institutes of Health (NIH)) "for their discovery of G-proteins and the role of these proteins in signal transduction in cells."[2] (A comprehensive description of the work that led to Gilman's Nobel Prize is presented in chapter 6.) Flashing his characteristic sardonic grin, Gilman stated,

> Later in the day when people started asking the usual canned questions about how it felt when the phone rang, I told them that I immediately secreted all the adrenaline I had and then started activating my receptor and my G-proteins to make more. That was the perfect answer from me. It was a wonderful day, an absolutely fabulous day. We had lunch in the conference room at the medical school and there was a huge assembly of faculty and staff in the afternoon. Kern [Wildenthal, president of the UT Southwestern Medical Center] was out of the country, but Bill Neaves [then dean of the medical school] had a dinner for us in the evening and a number of really close friends came in from out of town. It was a day to remember![1]

The Nobel Prize brings a definite cachet not only to the individual scientist, but also to the institution with which the scientist is affiliated (especially if the work being recognized was executed there, although such happy coincidence is not always the case). Thus, while Gilman's award-winning research was initiated at the University of Virginia in the early 1970s, he had been a faculty member at UT Southwestern since 1980 and was considered one of many "adopted Texans."

Cities and states, even entire countries, enjoy the spotlight of the Nobel Prize and are quick to celebrate when one of their own ascends to such coveted heights. No other award for human endeavor brings with it quite the

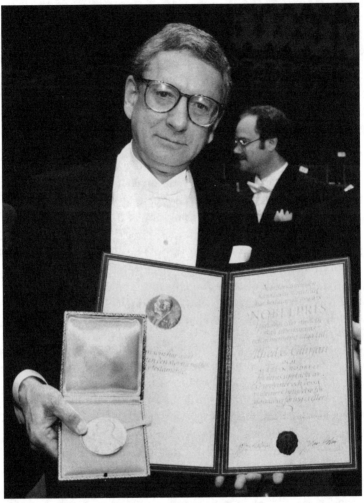

Alfred G. Gilman (left) and Martin Rodbell (right) at the 1994 Nobel Prize ceremonies in Stockholm. The pair was awarded the Physiology or Medicine Prize.

same level of prestige and distinction, and few if any stir feelings of such awe
in the general public. Harriet Zuckerman, author of *The Scientific Elite: Nobel
Laureates in the United States,* aptly summed up the status of the Prize when
she commented, "[it] is the gold standard by which all other scientific awards
are judged—[it is the] universal and instantly understood metaphor of
supreme achievement."[3]

Gilman's early morning call from Stockholm was, therefore, more than a
personal accolade. It was a defining moment in the history of a medical school

born just fifty years earlier in a city better recognized for its football team than its academic prowess, a city still recovering from the assassination of President John F. Kennedy, and one desperately trying to shake off its branding by the popular TV soap opera of the same name. To comprehend the significance of the coveted Nobel Prize, consider the following. There are over 2,000 colleges and universities in the U.S. (including 126 medical schools), not to mention numerous private research institutions. By 1997, nearly a century after the inception of the Nobel Prizes, scientists and scholars from just thirty-six American educational or research organizations had been so honored. Only fifteen U.S. institutions (all universities) have garnered four or more Prizes. Until the time of this writing UT Southwestern Medical Center at Dallas was the only medical school in the world with four Nobel Laureates. However, this unique distinction must be qualified in light of the award of two Nobel Prizes to Stanford University Medical School in 2006.

UT Southwestern's academic triumphs continued well beyond 1994. To mention just a smattering of these, the following year, Steven (Steve) McKnight, a native Texan and one of the youngest American scientists elected to membership of the U.S. National Academy of Sciences (the Academy), was recruited to the Department of Biochemistry, succeeding Joseph (Joe) Sambrook as the department chairman a few years later. Sambrook, another world-class scientist and a Fellow of the Royal Society of London (the British equivalent of the U.S. National Academy of Sciences) had moved to Australia, but not before he recruited Johann Deisenhofer to Southwestern Medical School in 1998. Eight months after he arrived in Dallas Deisenhofer became UT Southwestern's third Nobel laureate, joining Joseph Goldstein and Michael Brown. Eric N. Olson and Thomas C. Südhof (both destined for election to the U.S. National Academy of Sciences) were appointed to leadership positions in the school and Masashi Yanagisawa, Xiaodong Wang, Melanie Cobb, and David Russell would add to the growing list of UT Southwestern's membership in the elite U.S. National Academy. Finally, just a few months before this book went to press, Xiaodong Wang, a former graduate student and post-doctoral fellow at UT Southwestern and now professor of biochemistry and Howard Hughes Medical Institute Investigator, captured the prestigious Shaw Prize in Life Science and Medicine, a relatively recent award established by the Hong Kong-based Shaw Prize Foundation and already referred to as the "Nobel Prize of the East."

By 2006, seventeen resident faculty at the medical school had been elected to the U.S. National Academy (see Appendix), the highest honor to which any American scientist can realistically aspire. (To aspire to the Nobel Prize is most certainly not realistic!) Let's take a moment to consider this statistic. In 2003, the total active membership of the Academy (founded by President Abraham Lincoln in 1863) was over 2,300 individuals, representing the biological and economic sciences, astronomy, mathematics, geology, geophysics, physics, and engineering. Fewer than forty of the approximately 2,000 U.S. academic institutions can boast more than ten members of the Academy on their faculty. A free-standing medical school such as UT Southwestern can qualify for only about a third of the total membership positions, since it has no faculty representation in economics, astronomy, mathematics, geology, physics or engineering. By any reckoning, therefore, having seventeen faculty members at the Academy represents salutary institutional recognition. Indeed, in terms of the ratio of faculty elected to the Academy to total faculty size, UT Southwestern ranks fourth in the U.S.

The medical school in Dallas boasts impressive ranks in other metrics of academic excellence. The school ranks second in the U.S. in the ratio of Howard Hughes Investigatorships to total faculty. (The Howard Hughes Medical Institute, the largest private source of funds for biomedical research in the country, awards prestigious investigatorships to faculty members.) In terms of the impact of scientific papers published in biomedical literature from 1997–2001, UT Southwestern ranked in the top ten institutions in four of six scientific fields analyzed. Finally, UT Southwestern ranks in the top ten institutions in overall medical school faculty excellence, a measure based on multiple criteria, including surveys of medical school deans, competition for NIH research grants, competition for Howard Hughes Investigatorships, and election to prestigious organizations such as the Academy and its Institute of Medicine. Other institutions in the top ten include established stalwarts of biomedical excellence such as Harvard, Yale, and Johns Hopkins.

In 1996, UT Southwestern's rapid ascendancy to scientific prominence attracted the attention of the weekly journal *Science*. The journal quoted the late Maxwell Cowan, then vice-president and chief scientific officer of the Howard Hughes Medical Institute, as follows: "'UT Southwestern has moved into the

INSTITUTIONAL PROFILE

UT Southwestern: From Army Shacks to Research Elites

The November 29, 1996 issue of the weekly journal SCIENCE carried a piece on UT Southwestern.

front rank of medical schools in the last several years ... and it's the only school to have done so in the last decade.'"[4]

With over 1.5 million square feet of new research space on the spacious North Campus facility and a faculty comprised of over 1,300 physicians and scientists, UT Southwestern now casts a massive shadow over the fledgling organization spawned in crisis in 1943, an organization with no physical facility it could call its own, no financial infrastructure, and a rudimentary, largely part-time faculty.

Fueled by intense competition with the former Soviet Union, the Cold War years fostered unprecedented growth and prosperity for academically based biomedical research in the U.S. While UT Southwestern Medical Center at Dallas is by no means the only American medical school that accrued substantial financial and academic gains during this period, it is generally acknowledged that none other began with quite so little and few if any achieved quite so much in so short a time. What follows is the story of UT Southwestern's intellectual and physical transformation.

CHAPTER 2

EARLY MEDICAL EDUCATION AND RESEARCH IN THE UNITED STATES

The history of U.S. medical education and research has been extensively documented and does not bear detailed repetition here. But even a superficial analysis of the emergence of a medical school to a position of national prominence demands some general historical perspective.

American medicine, and in particular American biomedical research, occupies a hallowed position in the world. But such was not always the case. French clinical medicine enjoyed this exalted state during the first half of the 19th century, being succeeded by German academic medicine. In the U.S., medicine and medical education were nothing short of abysmal during most of the 19th century. In his scholarly work *Learning to Heal: The Development of American Medical Education*,[1] historian Kenneth Ludmerer presents an absorbing account of this moribund situation. During the Civil War (1861–65), "[t]he training and skills of the average doctor were hopelessly inadequate, even based on existing standards of the day."[1] The qualification of "existing standards" bears emphasis. In the mid-19th century, healing the sick and wounded was depressingly limited in every country in the world. Indeed, a sectarian movement founded in the U.S. by Samuel Thompson (1769–1843) opposed formal medical schooling and medical science (such as it was), embracing natural healing instead. Thompson, a product of a rural farming family, learned at an early age the pervasive "root and herb" practice popular in the 18th and early 19th centuries. Later he became an avid reader of the medical literature[2] and he and his follow Thompsonians argued, with much justification, that doctors were essentially useless, and suggested that the sick would be better off administering to themselves with herbs and other natural products.

During the Civil War "elementary techniques of physical examination such as measuring temperature ... were performed by [only] a small portion of ... physicians."[1] The use of basic medical instruments such as the stethoscope was

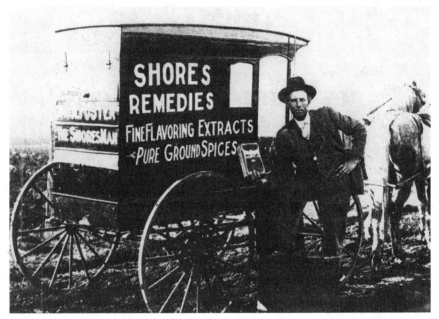

A traveling medicine man who pedaled his wares in the Dallas area circa 1900.

the exception rather than the rule, and antisepsis procedures had not yet been adopted. Indeed, the famous English surgeon Joseph Lister, often heralded as the father of antisepsis, was then still trying to convince his colleagues of the efficacy of washing their hands and of using carbolic acid to cleanse wounds. So it was standard practice for Union and Confederate army surgeons to poke their unwashed fingers into suppurating wounds and cursorily wipe their hands on their filthy aprons before repeating the procedure on another unfortunate soldier.

✳ ✳ ✳ ✳ ✳

Medical education in the U.S. didn't fare much better. To gain entry to a proprietary school (medical school at the time), candidates required nothing beyond an elementary school education. Literacy was not at all obligatory. These so-called institutions of learning were owned and operated by small groups of practicing doctors, primarily for economic gain. (Believe it or not, students were required to pay tuition to attend these bastions of higher education!) Facilities were typically rented space in which lectures could be delivered at minimal cost, often above a drugstore to which the new doctors could refer business. By the early 1860s several dozen of these proprietary schools existed in the country. The curriculum was entirely didactic, typically comprising daily lectures by "local experts" for two four-month terms. Doctors usually graduated without written examinations—what was the point if so many couldn't write?—and often had never touched a patient, witnessed a surgical procedure, or observed a birth.

A small number of ambitious men (there were no women doctors then) pursued alternative pathways to becoming physicians. Some opted to position themselves as an apprentice to a practicing doctor. While fine in theory, this apprenticeship system was dreadfully exploited. "Few preceptors made any effort to provide systematic instruction to their trainees, and even when they did, their efforts were usually hindered by the lack of books, equipment, and clinical resources, as well as their unfamiliarity with recent developments in medical knowledge. Many apprentices spent more time performing menial household chores for their preceptors than learning medicine."[1]

Some pursued an education in one of a small number of non-degree-granting private "medical schools" that provided clinical training exclusively during the summer months. But only the wealthy could afford to forgo gainful employment in the summer. Thus, far fewer of these existed than the proprietary schools. Others became so-called house pupils, the forerunners of the English housemen, residing (in house) in hospitals and assuming hands-on responsibility for the physical welfare of patients. This practice, too, was not widespread. However, those who opted for this mode of medical training became reasonably competent physicians, at least by the standards of those days. Indeed, "many former house pupils would later become leaders of the movement to upgrade clinical teaching in America."[1] Finally, some—almost exclusively members of the upper economic class—chose to study abroad in France and later Germany. From 1820–61, nearly 700 Americans studied medicine in Paris, and from 1870–1914, at least 10,000 studied in Vienna.[1]

Around the time of the Civil War, medical research was essentially unheard of in American medical schools. The handful of intellectually curious physicians bent on applying the scientific method to medical practice did so at their own expense and on their own time. "The same spirit of practicality—some would say anti-intellectualism—that pervaded other aspects of life in a [young] country still expanding its borders and conquering its terrain, penetrated the medical profession as well."[1] Given the pervasive dynamism and vigor that characterized the rapidly emerging United States of America, however, reform in medical practice and education was inevitable. Like most transformations, this came about slowly—and often painfully. But importantly, increasing numbers of those who attended the authoritative German medical schools in the late 19th century became keenly motivated to emulate what they'd learned in Europe and ultimately "came to form the faculties at Johns Hopkins, Harvard, Michigan, Cornell, and other medical schools that were the first to introduce modern teaching methods in the United States. They were also responsible for establishing America's reputation in medical research."[1] Though small in number, this band of doctors was inspired by the sophistication of German laboratory-based medical science, and sought to identify themselves as medical academicians rather than medical practitioners. They "sought intellectual distinction rather than monetary rewards."[1]

This was easier said than done. The infrastructure to support academic careers in medicine was essentially non-existent. Additionally, anyone who went to the trouble and expense of traveling to Germany for modern medical training and then returned with an academic "bug" in his ear was considered somewhat eccentric—to say the least. When William H. Welch, the renowned professor of Pathology at Johns Hopkins University (whose many distinguished protégés were referred to as the "Welsh rarebits"), announced his intention to occupy that academic position upon his return from Germany, his closest friend, a prominent practicing physician in New York, was shocked to the extent that their friendship was irrevocably fractured.

In short, "[i]n the 1870s and 1880s ... a handful of dedicated, pioneering medical scientists managed to secure and maintain academic positions by virtue of the great economic and personal sacrifices they were willing to make. The few professional positions available were seized by those willing to overlook meager salaries, arduous working conditions and suboptimal facilities, for the opportunity to devote themselves to teaching and research."[1]

❋ ❋ ❋ ❋ ❋

Following the Civil War, the American university system made a radical departure from the didactic and pedantic dogmatism of the old-fashioned college system. The university emerged as the educational vehicle for *all* intellectual endeavors, including medicine. This in turn had a significant impact on medical teaching. "By the turn of the century the university was medical education's greatest friend and protector—the provider of a secure institutional home, a source of financial support, and a reservoir of intellectual encouragement. The American university provided a prominent place for medicine in the country's system of higher education."[1]

These changes were gradual of course. Immediately after the Civil War, "the proprietary schools continued to provide the same superficial course of lectures [and] the casual admission and graduation requirements of the antebellum period—continued essentially unchanged. Among better trained physicians, the influence of the [older] French clinical school with its emphasis on careful observation rather than scientific enquiry was strong, fostering a continuing skepticism about the utility of scientific knowledge in clinical practice."[1] But the influence of the newer German school and its emphasis on clinical research was growing, and its alliance with the American university was increasing.

A clash was inevitable between adherents to the older, largely clinically based French and the more modern, academically focused German medical cultures. It first surfaced between 1871–93 at Harvard, Penn, Michigan, and Johns Hopkins, where young, energetic, and forward-looking minds collided with older, entrenched, and politically powerful leaders. The final outcome, however, was never in doubt. Harvard Medical School is a particularly instructive example of how determined reform can turn an antiquated system on its head.

In the late 1860s admission to Harvard Medical School was open to essentially anyone who could afford the fee. "Only twenty percent of the students held college degrees, and one faculty member estimated in 1870 that over half the students could not write."[1] Sweeping change came when a dynamic educational reformist was elected president. Charles William Eliot was a member of a prominent Boston Brahmin family and was culturally and philosophically dedicated to public service. Under his forty-year administration, Harvard grew from a small college with various attached professional schools into a great modern university. "The elective system was extended, the curriculum was enriched through the addition of new courses, written examinations were required [and] the faculty was enlarged.... Increased entrance requirements prevailed both in the college and in the professional schools, which Eliot reformed and revitalized."[3]

Eliot had observed both the French and German medical educational systems while studying mathematics and chemistry in Europe. Upon becoming Harvard's president, he made the reform of medical education a priority. In his first report delivered in 1870, he acerbically commented, "[t]he ignorance and general incompetency of the average graduate of American Medical Schools at the time when he receives the degree which turns him loose upon the community, is something horrible to contemplate."[1]

Eliot personally assumed the chairmanship of the medical school faculty— a most unusual move by a university president—and retained this position for the next forty years! Meetings of this body were not mere "conflict between elite and ordinary physicians, but a civil war within the ranks of the elite."[1] Senior and powerful members of the Harvard faculty such as Oliver Wendell Holmes (also a noted writer and the father of the renowned American jurist of the same name) and Henry Jacob Bigelow (the famous Harvard professor of Surgery who promoted the use of anesthesia in American medical practice) questioned why Eliot was encouraging reforms that would discard a system that in their view had been successful for eighty years. " 'The reason', Eliot answered in an immortalized reply, was quite simple: 'there is a new President.' "[1]

Eliot brought about vigorous change at Harvard Medical School. The curriculum was increased in breadth and depth, and was extended from two to three years. Subjects were taught in a logical sequence and notably included the laboratory sciences. In addition to anatomy, students were now instructed in chemistry, pathology, physiology, and histology. In 1880 Harvard made a fourth year of training optional. But within a dozen years the fourth year became mandatory—a curriculum that endures to this day. Significantly, by 1900 a bachelor degree from a university was required for admission. The days of illiteracy among aspiring physicians were gone forever and medicine was no longer a trade of dubious means.

In the early 1890s, the Johns Hopkins Medical School also underwent drastic change. Described as "the most spectacular innovation in the history of American medical education.... Hopkins became the envy of every forward-looking medical school in the country."[1] The school instituted rigorous admission standards, established a four-year curriculum divided equally into basic science and clinical training, and recruited an outstanding faculty. It erected new buildings equipped with state-of-the-art facilities including research laboratories, and acquired its own university hospital. Importantly, following explicit instruction from its benefactor Johns Hopkins, the medical school was integrated into the university organization, an alliance that was soon to become the benchmark of any quality medical school in the U.S.

✳ ✳ ✳ ✳ ✳

By the turn of the 20th century, medical education in the U.S. was modernizing rapidly. This reform was accelerated by the now famous (or infamous, depending on one's viewpoint) Flexner Report, *Medical Education in the United States and Canada*.[4] Abraham Flexner was not a physician; he was an educator. Born in 1866, Flexner became a secondary school teacher and eventually school principal in Louisville, Kentucky, positions he retained for nineteen years. Following graduate study at Harvard and the University of Berlin, he joined the Carnegie Foundation for the Advancement of Teaching. This activist foundation sponsored a comprehensive study of medical education for which Flexner journeyed to medical schools across the U.S. and Canada.

His report, issued in 1910, denounced the "scandalous conditions" in proprietary schools, praised quality medical schools, and castigated inferior ones. "To Flexner, only one type of medical school was acceptable: university

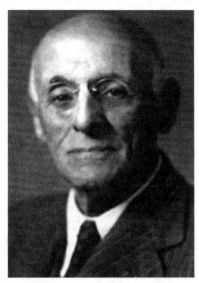

Abraham Flexner (1866–1959) was an American educator who is credited with reforming medical education in the United States and Canada. Flexner also founded the Institute for Advanced Study at Princeton University in 1930 and served as its first director.

schools, with large full-time faculties and a vigorous commitment to research."[1] The report received enormous attention both in the academic community and among the informed public. "[The report] made instant headlines, and newspapers accepted its conclusions as gospel."[1]

Why did the results of an academically based study strike such a responsive chord with the American public? The answer is straightforward. The Flexner Report promoted increased public awareness that good medical education and research generated good health care. "His report—and later Flexner himself—helped persuade the public that it was in its own interest to support medical schools generously."[1] Flexner took care to emphasize the staggering financial requirements of modern medical education; his advocacy contributed substantially to the promotion of philanthropic support for U.S. medical schools, as increasing numbers of patrons keen on modernizing medical education and research came to realize that these were expensive endeavors. Regardless of these salutary efforts, by the beginning of the World War II only a minority of U.S. medical schools (most definitely not including UT Southwestern) were able to meet the financial demands required to move to and remain in the top tier.

In the early 20th century, the philanthropy that so greatly benefited American higher education was fueled by a period of huge national economic prosperity. Wealthy foundations such as the General Education Board (founded in 1902 by John D. Rockefeller, Sr.), the Rockefeller Foundation, and the Carnegie Corporation were vital to this endeavor and "participated in the philanthropic enterprise on a heretofore unimagined scale."[1] From 1902–34, a mere nine foundations donated $154 million to medical schools (a sum that roughly translates to about $17 billion in 2005). Private donors and progressive state legislatures donated even larger amounts. In many cases, wealthy patrons made contributions "that allowed the course of their favored school to be turned around almost overnight,"[1] a state of mind that now characterizes American academia in general. Later chapters of this book will reveal the profound influence of philanthropy on the development of UT Southwestern at several crucial periods.

By the 1920s, medical education in the U.S. had matured close to the level we see today. In 1934, the first of a protracted harvest of Nobel Prizes to be awarded to faculty at U.S. medical schools was given to George Whipple of Rochester University in Medicine and George Minot and William Murphy at the Harvard Medical School for discoveries that facilitated the treatment of anemia with liver extracts.

CHAPTER 3

THE BIRTH OF A MEDICAL SCHOOL IN DALLAS

"I remember that in January of 1951 I got into my Kaiser, which was the car we had then, with my wife and my daughter, and we drove from New Haven, Connecticut to Dallas, stopping off in Washington to visit friends. When we arrived in Dallas on January 8, I said to my wife, Muriel: 'I would like to see the medical school before we find some place to stay.' So we located Maple Avenue and Oak Lawn Boulevard, which was the address I'd been given. There was a filling station on the corner and I asked the attendant where the medical school was. He gestured toward the railroad crossing down Oak Lawn. So I drove there and looked around, but I couldn't see anything that looked like a medical school. I went back and told the attendant that I didn't see any medical school, just a bunch of shacks—and scattered garbage. 'That's the medical school,' he said emphatically. So I drove back again and examined the army-style barracks more closely. That was indeed the medical school. The shacks had been transported as prefabricated structures and assembled there. They were just placed on the ground—there were no foundations dug. If the weather became cold the school would have to shut down because there was no warming system. It was steaming hot in the summer and the floors, which were wooden, started decaying and were full of holes—and so was the ceiling. The students used to joke that someone walking across the floor would fall into one of the holes and disappear forever.

The school was located right behind the old Parkland Hospital then located on Maple Avenue. The hospital had been built in the early 1920s and was probably out-moded at the time that it opened! The students used to call the emergency room the black hole of Calcutta. It was a very obsolete institution. So this was Southwestern Medical School—Parkland Hospital and a bunch of barracks located on Oak Lawn and Maple Avenues!"[1]

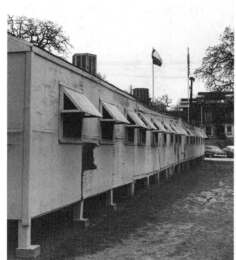
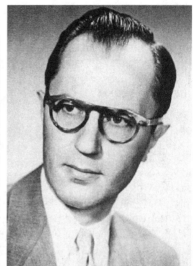
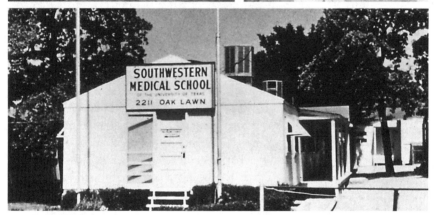

Temporary shacks on Oak Lawn Avenue donated by the U.S. Army housed the Southwestern Medical College of the Southwest Medical Foundation, and later the University of Texas Southwestern Medical School. This is the sight that greeted Don Seldin (above right) when he first arrived in Dallas in early January 1951.

Such was Donald W. Seldin's introduction to what was then called *Southwestern Medical School of the University of Texas*, a name that was changed in 1954 to *The University of Texas Southwestern Medical School*, and again in 1972 to *The University of Texas Health Sciences Center at Dallas*. In 1987 the institution reverted to almost precisely its 1954 designation when it was labeled *The University of Texas Southwestern Medical Center at Dallas*. The school's first moniker, *The*

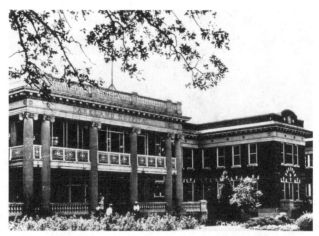

The second Parkland Hospital opened its doors at Maple and Oak Lawn Avenues in 1913 on a 23-acre patch of land and held 100 patients. The city of Dallas spent $112,000 on the facility, which was hailed as "one of the best equipped institutions of its kind in the Southwest."

Southwestern Medical College of the Southwestern Medical Foundation was adopted in 1943. Throughout most of the text I have adopted the now commonly used "UT Southwestern" to identify the institution in its contemporary mode.

Not surprisingly, the frequent name changes did little to promote brand recognition. So, when Michael Brown and Joseph Goldstein won the school's first Nobel Prizes in 1984 (discussed in chapter 7), the national and even the local press credited no less than eight different academic institutions in Texas with the award, including The University of Dallas (unrelated to the University of Texas System) and Southwestern University (a small undergraduate institution located in Georgetown, Central Texas). Even as recently as the early 1990s I was amazed by the frequency with which people to whom I mentioned Southwestern assumed that I was talking about the Southwestern Bell telephone company! Mercifully, this confusion has all but evaporated—largely because Southwestern Bell changed *its* name!

* * * * *

The origin of the Southwestern Medical College of the Southwestern Medical Foundation is deeply rooted with a single individual, Edward Henry Cary, a physician and a man of extraordinary vision and purpose who, like Donald Seldin a half century later, harbored lofty ambitions of medical care, medical education and medical research in the southwestern United States.

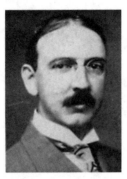

Edward Henry Cary (1872–1953) arrived in Dallas in 1890. He attended medical school at Bellevue Hospital Medical College in New York from 1895 to 1898, then returned to Dallas in 1901 to set up a practice in ophthalmology.

Edward Henry Cary was born in 1872 in the rural town of Chunnenugee, Alabama. His father, a Confederate soldier who was captured by the Union Army and returned to his Alabama plantations after his release, died when Cary was an infant. In Cary's biography, *More Than Armies: The Story of Edward H. Cary, MD*,[2] Booth Mooney informs us that when fourteen-year-old Cary's older brothers left Alabama to seek their fortunes, the young teenager "began his formal business career by becoming manager of his mother's two cotton plantations."[2] As a youth Cary suffered a distressing visual problem. When he read by candlelight his eyes often flickered in rhythm with the candles, causing him considerable frustration, at times prompting him to wonder despairingly whether he might go blind. He visited numerous doctors, but to no avail. It was this infirmity that prompted his interest in becoming a physician.

When Cary's brother Albert Powell Cary moved to Dallas to enter a dental supply business, he frequently urged young Edward to join him. Eventually, at the age of eighteen, Cary shelved his dreams of becoming a doctor and joined Albert, arriving in Dallas on New Year's Eve of 1890. "Edward promptly fell in love with the city in whose future development he was to play so prominent a role."[2] Dallas, at the end of 1890, was already becoming one of the most important cities in Texas. Named in 1845 by founder John Neely Bryan in honor of U.S. Vice President George Mifflin Dallas, the city was one of the largest in the largest state in the Union. Cary was excited by what he encountered. "Dallas, he felt … was a place where important people did important things.... The people were amazingly friendly. Folks had been friendly in Alabama too, but this Texas friendliness had a breezy, casual air that was quite different."[2]

The history of medicine and medical care in Dallas is not dissimilar from that in most frontier towns in the United States of America. It is reported that

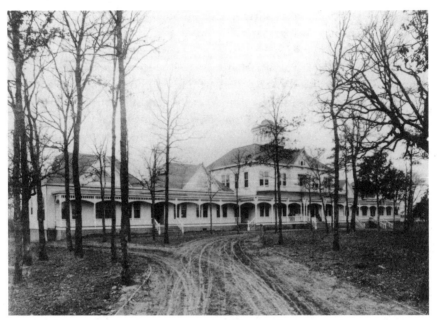

The first Parkland Hospital was located at the same site as the second facility (see page 19). It opened in 1894 and cost $40,000 to build.

the first resident physician, "a Dr. Calder, was attacked and killed by native inhabitants in 1842 near the present intersection of Lomo Alto and Lemmon Avenue, a year after John Neely Bryan established Dallas."[3] By 1870, Dallas had a population of about 40,000. A few years later, three local physicians opened the first "hospital" to treat indigent patients, requiring only that the city reimburse them for their supplies. A new hospital was erected in 1874 in a single-room house (twenty-five by fifty feet) with an adjoining kitchen and privy. Five years later, following complaints lodged in the *Dallas Herald*, the city added a building (eighteen square feet) for female patients and purchased $28.50 worth of surgical instruments.[3]

Commenting on the general state of health care and the regulation of medical practice in Texas in the late 20th century, John Chapman noted the pervasive existence of so-called second-floor letter drops located in low-rent areas of Dallas that conferred an MD degree by return post in exchange for a letter of intent and a fee of fifteen dollars.[4] Dallas citizens voted for a $40,000 bond for a new hospital in 1893 and the following year the first Parkland Hospital (named for the surrounding wooded park) opened its doors on a thirty-six-acre site just outside the city limits, at the intersection of Oak Lawn and Maple

Avenues.[3] The city of Dallas purchased an ambulance for $500 and a horse to pull it was bought two years later. Rubber tires were acquired in 1899 "as a necessary act of humanity."[14]

Shortly after his arrival in Dallas Cary joined his older brother's dental supply business (which now included medical and hospital supplies) traveling extensively in the southwest to meet customers and court new business. As a youth he'd been somewhat shy, but now "he grew a moustache and gained confidence in himself."[2] In short, Cary enjoyed working for his brother. He was earning a respectable living and he took pleasure in the city and its people. His eyes, however, continued to worsen and more and more, "he wanted to know the truth about whatever caused him to undergo periodic attacks of near-blindness.... Slowly, inevitably, the boyhood dream of becoming a doctor returned to him. [Perhaps] [t]hat would be the way to find the truth."[2]

But where to attend medical school? On his business trips, Cary had seen enough of late 19th century medical schools in Texas, Oklahoma, and Louisiana to know that he did not "want any part of this misnamed medical education. There could only be one school for him. That was Bellevue Hospital Medical College"[2] in New York, then considered the finest medical school in the country.

❊ ❊ ❊ ❊ ❊

Bellevue Medical College boasted an outstanding department of ophthalmology, and from Cary's first exposure to the discipline, "ophthalmology became the center of his existence."[2] After graduating in 1898, Cary interned at the famous Eye Infirmary at Bellevue and was soon "looked upon by other members of his profession in New York as a young man going somewhere."[2] It was at the Eye Infirmary that he was properly fitted with glasses that "corrected the astigmatic condition which had been the basis of his life-time eye distress. Cary saw before him in New York the promise of all that any doctor could hope to attain. Flattering offers of a professorship in the Polyclinic, a pioneer postgraduate medical school in New York, were placed before him soon after the completion of his internship in January 1901."[2] But, as is so often the case, unforeseen events changed the course of his life. His brother Albert died leaving their mother uncared for and Cary was required to return to Dallas to fend for his mother and to settle his older sibling's affairs.

"Cary examined carefully the medical wilderness that he found Texas to be in the year 1901. There were plenty of doctors. But few of them had been scientifically trained. Too many were products of the inferior medical schools that had continued to multiply."[2] Cary established what he believed would be a temporary medical practice while his brother's affairs were put in order. The practice flourished, especially in ophthalmology (then a specialty with limited available expertise in Dallas). Still, Cary did not plan to remain in the city. He "was determined that he must both practice and teach his profession"[2] in New York, not some remote corner of the southwest. His return to the northeast, however, was continually delayed. On top of the imperative to settle his brother's estate, his ailing widowed mother, having moved to Dallas to be with Albert, enjoyed living there. Providentially, within a short time of opening his practice Cary became "the central figure in a controversy that divided the city's medical profession into two bitterly opposite camps and [eventually] the idea of moving back to New York went out of his mind for all time."[2]

* * * * *

Not long before Cary returned to Dallas, Charles McDaniel Rosser, a twenty-seven-year-old doctor, established himself in the city as a practicing physician. Rosser was no average town doctor. A man with substantial intellectual aspirations, he enjoyed public speaking and was often quoted in local newspapers. Rosser orated on all manner of topics, including cultism, chiropractors, and Christian Scientism, and is said to have once delivered a talk about overspecialization in medicine, in rhyme! John Fordtran, a former faculty member at UT Southwestern and a scholar of early medicine in Dallas, noted that Rosser even wrote poetry related to medicine.[4]

Rosser considered himself a cut above the average practicing doctor, and disapproved that Dallas doctors "were taking on artificial airs. A silk top hat and a Prince Albert coat were everyday regalia for Dallas doctors [and Rosser] was compelled to borrow money for a handsome horse and an elegant rig. A doctor without these wouldn't be appreciated."[4] But Rosser's attitude stemmed from more than mere eccentricity. He was an ambitious man who, when serving as Health Officer for the City of Dallas in 1892, campaigned aggressively for a new hospital, pointing out that while other Texas hospitals could accommodate several hundred patients, the Dallas hospital could manage only forty-two. Eventually he persuaded Mayor Ben E. Cabell to announce an open meeting to consider starting a medical school in the city. On August 15, 1900, the following notice appeared in the *Dallas Morning News*.[5]

At the request of a large number of physicians of Dallas and Oak Cliff we respectfully announce that a meeting will be held in the Council Chamber of the city hall on Thursday, August 16, at 8:30 pm, for the purpose of taking the necessary preliminary steps to establish a med-

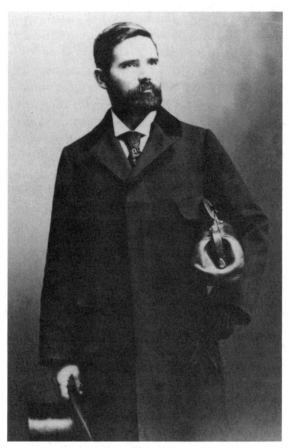

Charles McDaniel Rosser (1862–1945) studied medicine at the University of Louis-ville. He established a practice in Waxahachie, Texas, then moved to Dallas in 1889.

ical college in Dallas. All regular physicians in good standing are invited to be present and to aid in organizing a college.

Rosser's persuasive manner notwithstanding, it is unclear what events or circumstances prompted the mayor of Dallas to issue his proclamation. John
Chapman commented that "the letter-drop diplomas were a disgrace to any
place, and Mayor Cabell may have concluded that the best way to get rid of
them would be to provide some sounder competition. Or, he may simply have
decided that a medical school was a proper appurtenance of a big city (population 42,638 in 1900)."[6] Fifty-four physicians attended the meeting—seven to
support the idea and forty-seven to fight it. The discussion was spirited and at
one point Rosser assailed his fellow physicians about their lack of enthusiasm.

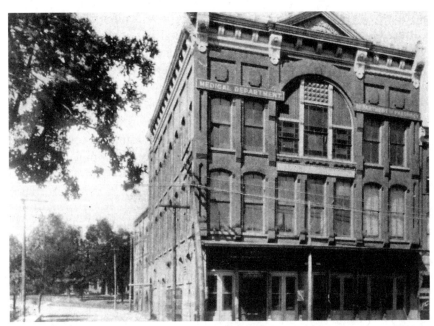

The Medical Department of the University of Dallas relocated to a building on S. Ervay Street in Dallas after the original medical college at Temple Emanu-el was destroyed by fire in 1902.

"Medical students are bright fellows [note the lack of consideration for women doctors] and one who assumes to teach them will have his measure taken," Rosser admonished the assembled audience. "I tell you now, not as a threat but as a matter for information, there is going to be a medical college in Dallas. There are a number of ambitious and qualified doctors variously located throughout the state who, if invited to faculty membership will come, and when you get more competition than you know what to do with, don't blame me."[4]

Despite considerable opposition the minority opinion prevailed. On November 19, 1900, a new medical college opened its doors in an abandoned synagogue, the old Temple Emanu-el, on Commerce Street, near what is now the Adolphus Hotel in downtown Dallas. (In 1902, this facility was destroyed in a fire and relocated to S. Ervay Street). Rosser was the first dean. Displaying remarkable ingenuity, the founders of the school obtained a charter for the University of Dallas Medical Department, even though at the time there was no such thing as the University of Dallas! Hospital affiliation was achieved through the Good Samaritan Hospital, originally a fourteen-room house purchased by Rosser and his colleagues in 1900. (Even though the Flexner Report would not be published for a decade, university affiliation had become important to medical schools—without it, survival was unlikely.)

At its inception, the combined staff and student population of the University of Dallas Medical Department was about seventy. A special issue of the journal *Legacies* (a history journal for Dallas and North Central Texas) published in 1993 provides a charming picture of the new school in an interview with its sole female student, Hallie Earle (she remained the only female student until 1910, and one of only 1,200 female medical students counted in the U.S. Census of 1900). On October 22, 1904, Hallie wrote home: "Yesterday Prof. Brooks of Waco was in Dallas and came around—and what do you think—Dr. Cary told him that it would be a chase between a red-headed boy and myself as to who would be leader in the sophomore class. I was perfectly thunderstruck."[7]

Celebration of the new medical school was short lived. Chapman notes that "within two months of the opening of the school a faculty insurrection developed"[6] and a splinter group split off to start the rival Dallas Medical College. "Just what all the difficulties were about has not been stated in the clearest terms."[6] According to Booth Mooney, "[The problems were] based primarily … on love of the *status quo*. The established doctors in Dallas liked things the way they were. Some petty professional or personal jealousies undoubtedly were involved, as was a certain narrowness of vision in medical circles at the time."[2] John Fordtran wrote: "Animosity towards the medical school [the University of Dallas Medical Department] was fierce … [and] Rosser was the focal point of much of the antagonism."[4]

Cary and Rosser became acquainted soon after Cary's arrival in Dallas. Rosser, impressed by his younger colleague's credentials and strong academic bent, courted Cary to join the faculty of his new medical college. But Cary was hesitant. He still wanted to return to New York, and recognized that "a connection with the school would not make his professional path easier in Dallas.… Opposition to the school was strongly entrenched and was capable of causing difficulty for a newcomer."[2]

Mooney recounts that one night in 1901 Rosser and Cary talked into the wee hours, downing "pot after pot of coffee while they gravely discussed the opposition to the school. They agreed that some of their elders were barely capable of doing a urinalysis, no matter how pleasant their social company might be. They deplored the prejudice felt by the unschooled toward the schooled. Rosser placed before Cary a glowing picture of the possibilities open to the school, urging him to take over the chair of ophthalmology."[2] By the time the sun had began to rise, Cary was persuaded. " 'I'll do it,' he said at the end of the all-night session. 'I'm with you.' "[2]

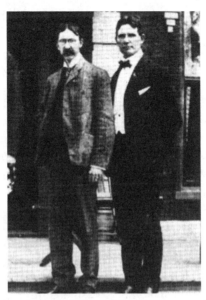

Charles Rosser (right) and Edward Cary (left) became acquainted soon after Cary arrived in Dallas.

No sooner was Cary's appointment made public than he encountered the wrath of the school's entrenched opposition. "They did not like the thought of such a man as Cary lending his talents to the school [and] they told him so."[2] The situation was further complicated by the emergence of warring factions within the school, resulting in defections to the Dallas Medical College. Such complexities notwithstanding, Cary was generally viewed as a moderate, as a man who listened and mediated. In time, "the various factions came to regard Cary as the one man to resolve their differences. They could not deal amicably with one another, but they could deal with Cary."[2] In due course Cary succeeded Rosser as dean—a far cry from his aspirations to practice academic medicine in New York City.

Edward Cary was precisely what the new medical school needed. He was dynamic, energetic, determined, and tough; in short, an optimistic visionary and a formidable leader. He divided the school's 120 students into four classes and ruthlessly pruned out weakness, cutting the senior class down to just four students. "The first time a leading local physician, one who liked better than anything else to make orations before as many people as possible, appeared before the new senior class, he stormed out of the lecture room to offer his resignation. 'It's a waste of time,' he fumed to Cary. 'I simply will not come out here to talk to four damn fools.' 'Isn't it better,' Cary rejoined, 'to talk to four damn fools than to a hundred and twenty?'"[2] In 1901, its first year of operation, the University of Dallas Medical Department graduated fifteen doctors. In 1903, however, Cary awarded just three diplomas. He considered the fourth senior unqualified. "[Cary's] energy, enthusiasm, toughness, determination, and personality were outstanding."[4]

Soon after becoming dean of the new medical school, Cary attended the 1903 annual convention of the American Medical Association (AMA) in New Orleans. There he learned of the Association's firm intention to forever squelch the proprietary schools. Indeed, the president of the AMA predicted that within five years, no U.S. medical school without university affiliation would survive. Opportunities to find an academic home for the fledgling University of Dallas Medical Department were limited, however. The University of Texas at Austin already had a Medical Branch in Galveston, and no university in the country then had formal affiliation with more than one medical school.

On the train ride back from New Orleans a colleague suggested that Cary consider affiliating with Baylor University, a Baptist institution with a solid academic reputation located on the banks of the Brazos River in Waco, Texas. An associate of Cary's introduced him to George W. Truett, "the powerful and widely respected pastor of the First Baptist Church in Dallas and later president of the Baptist World Alliance,"[2] who had challenged Dallasites to build a "great humanitarian hospital,"[2] a plea that led to the construction of the Texas Baptist Memorial Sanitarium in 1909. Subsequent events notwithstanding, Cary and Truett remained life-long friends.

With Truett's help, Cary met with senior officials at Baylor University. John Chapman wrote: "Without bias with respect to creeds, Cary adopted a very canny approach to the problem. Baylor University was not only the oldest but probably also the largest, as well as the nearest, of the potential guardians. Furthermore, the Baptist denomination in Dallas was large, evangelical, and potentially well-to-do. Baylor, therefore, appeared to be a reasonable choice; and Cary set about arranging the adoption of his medical school." Discussions moved swiftly and decisively, and before 1903 was out the University of Dallas Medical Department became the Baylor University Medical College. While attempts to merge the University of Dallas Medical Department and the rival Dallas Medical College had failed the year before, Cary was able to persuade some of the rebel faculty to join Baylor University Medical College. In 1909, a new college building (Ramseur Hall) was erected, and in 1921, the Texas Baptist Memorial Sanitarium was renamed Baylor University Hospital to emphasize its relationship with the medical school. In 1922 Baylor University acquired East Dallas City Hall from the city of Dallas, and in 1932 it reopened as Edward H. Cary Hall to accommodate expanding needs in the medical and dental schools.

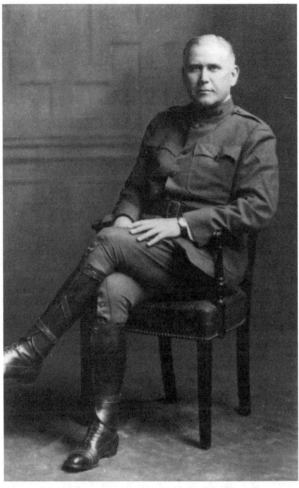

George Washington Truett (1867–1944). Under his leadership the First Baptist Church grew into the largest church in the world at that time, and he served as president of the Baptist World Alliance from 1934–1939. Truett introduced Cary to officials at Baylor University in Waco and the two remained life-long friends.

❋ ❋ ❋ ❋ ❋

Cary's efforts at promoting medical education in Dallas were advanced when he and Rosser convinced the famous Viennese orthopedic surgeon Adolf Lorenz to visit following the 1903 AMA convention. Lorenz agreed to a two-day visit but ended up spending a week at the Good Samaritan Hospital, conducting clinics for patients from all over Texas and beyond. His

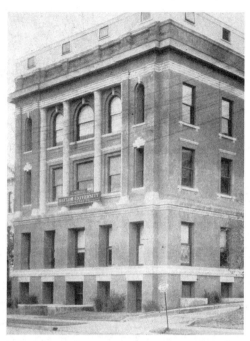

Ramseur Science Hall opened in 1909. Classes in the Baylor University College of Medicine and Dentistry were taught here for a period.

celebrity attracted the attention of civic leaders and promoted Cary's crusade for university affiliation for the Medical Department of the University of Dallas.[8]

As a historical aside, it is noteworthy that in 1903 yet another group of local physicians inaugurated a third medical school, called the Texas College of Physicians and Surgeons. When, later that year, the trustees of Southwestern University in Georgetown, Texas persuaded the four founding physicians of the Texas College of Physicians and Surgeons to establish their medical school as a department of Southwestern University, Southwestern University Medical College was founded. A short-lived institution that closed its doors in 1915, it was one of the many victims of Abraham Flexner's critical evaluation of American and Canadian medical schools. But for a brief period Dallas (with a population of a mere 40,000) had three medical schools — and a fourth was located in nearby Fort Worth, the Fort Worth School of Medicine having been organized in 1894. To be sure, whatever else its shortcomings, North Texas was no intellectual backwater as far as medical education was concerned.

Flexner's report on medical education included an incisive analysis of the fiscal state of medical schools. He noted: "There are in the United States and Canada fifty-six schools whose total annual available resources are below $10,000 each ... so small a sum that the endeavor to do anything substantial with it is of course futile."[7] In 1910, the income of Baylor University Medical College was $7,735. This pithy sum was derived exclusively from student tuition, as the affiliation agreement did not include financial support from the parent university in Waco. The budget at Southwestern Medical School was equally paltry. Flexner's comments on these schools were scathing. After grudgingly praising the University of Texas Medical Branch in Galveston, he wrote the following about the other Texas medical schools:

> The other ... schools are without resources, without ideals and without facilities, though at Baylor the conjunction of hospital and laboratory might be made effective if large sums, specifically applicable to medical education, were at hand—which is not, however, the case. There is no indication on the face of things that any of the three inferior schools can live through the dry period to the opportunities of the future.... The state is badly overcrowded with just the kind of doctor that they are engaged in producing. Should the loopholes in the present state standard be stopped up, all three would quickly disappear.[9]

✳ ✳ ✳ ✳ ✳

Cary continued to function as dean of the beleaguered Baylor University Medical College, though as he became increasingly more active in local, state, and regional medical affairs he had less and less to devote to the school. Flexner's caustic verdict notwithstanding, at the start of World War I Baylor University Medical College enjoyed an expanded student body and a Class A academic rating. Believing that his seventeen years of work had succeeded in solidly establishing the medical school, Cary ultimately resigned as dean (retaining the title of dean emeritus) to devote more time to his medical practice and to "execute ambitious plans that had been growing in his thoughts."[2] He erected the first Dallas skyscraper, a Medical Arts Building with physician's offices, and became a man of substantial financial means. Cary became increasingly more involved in local and regional medical politics, and in 1919 he was elected president of the Southern Medical Association. In 1932, his national visibility led him to his election as president of the AMA. "During his term of office Cary traveled 99,190 miles on the official business of the organization, and he was away from his home 340 days out of the two-year period."[2] During this entire time he served as dean

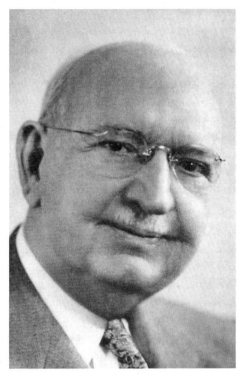

Edward Cary as a senior figure in Dallas medical affairs.

emeritus of Baylor Medical School and as chairman of the institution's administrative board. But Baylor University Medical College didn't fare as well as its founder. Difficult times ensued, and by 1938 the place was in dire financial straits. Around that time in fact, the executive vice-president warned that the medical school in Dallas would likely lose its Class A academic standing.

Despite his busy practice and his involvement with regional and national medical affairs, Cary continued to devote time and energy to improving medical education, practice, and research in Texas, indeed the entire Southwest. " 'The preceding half-century,' he pointed out, 'had seen the development of such outstanding medical centers as Johns Hopkins, the Cornell Center, Northwestern [and] the Mayo Foundation.' "[2] Why not a great medical center in Dallas? Recognizing the financial and logistical challenges that such an enterprise would entail, in 1939 he and a group of Dallas business associates founded the Southwestern Medical Foundation, a private organization devoted to promoting health care, research, and education in the southwestern U.S. The Foundation's charter stated:

It is formed for the establishment of facilities and clinics in the study of the causes, the prevention, and the cure of diseases of the minds and bodies of needy persons residing in the southwestern section of the United States and elsewhere, and for the development and training of laboratory workers, physicians and nurses in the treatment of diseased persons, in the study of individual and community hygiene, and in promoting public health, and in medical research.[10]

A handsome brochure published in 1943 further elaborated the foundation's philosophy. "The Board of Trustees of the Southwestern Medical Foundation secured a charter in 1939 for the perpetuation of medical education and scientific research in the Southwest. We believe firmly that through the accumulation of funds the progress already made in scientific medicine in the City of Dallas can be stimulated and developed to bring about one of the truly Great Medical Centers, similar to the few located in the North and East."[11]

Cary was supported in this medical crusade by a group of prominent Dallas businessmen that included Karl Hoblitzelle, president of Interstate Circuit, Inc. (a theater chain) and chairman of the Board of Republic National Bank; Fred Florence, president of Republic National Bank; E. R. Brown, president of Magnolia Petroleum and a director of the Federal Reserve Bank of Dallas; and Herbert Marcus, founder of the Neiman Marcus chain. Cary served as president of the foundation until his death in 1953.

✳ ✳ ✳ ✳ ✳

In the fall of 1941, Cary saw an opportunity to put his new enterprise to work. He approached Baylor University with plans for the Southwestern Medical Foundation to manage the financially beleaguered medical school in Dallas. Once again discussions moved swiftly and favorably, and in the spring of 1942, the foundation and the Baylor trustees signed a ninety-nine-year contract that yielded responsibility for operating the Baylor School of Medicine and College of Dentistry to the Southwestern Medical Foundation. But almost as soon as the agreement was signed Baylor's Board of Trustees voiced concerns about its nonsectarian wording. It is said that at the time that he established the foundation, Cary consulted with the trustees of the Rockefeller Foundation in New York, who cautioned him to avoid sectarian affiliations. In fact, Cary once categorically stated that "medicine has never secured funds for its maximum development under strictly denominational auspices, hence the creation of a Southwestern Medical Foundation to perpetuate education and scientific research in an assured nonsectarian environment."[2] Thus, under the terms of the contract, the school would no longer be identified with the Baptist church. Members of

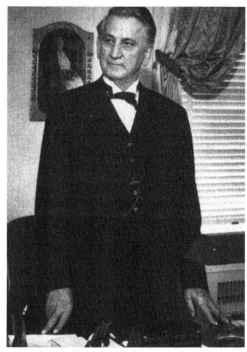

Pat Morris Neff (1871–1952) served as president of Baylor University, and as governor of Texas for two terms. A strict educator and careful financial administrator, he brought Baylor out of debt in the 1930s into a period of growth in the 1940s. During his tenure as president, enrollment at the university and the university endowment increased considerably. Despite these successes, many Baylor supporters viewed Neff as too rigid a disciplinarian who lacked a modern approach to education.

the foundation had argued that this provision was essential if the medical school was to be able to raise funds on an ongoing basis.[12]

It is unclear precisely when the nonsectarian issue surfaced. Regardless, on April 27, 1943, the Baylor University board voted to annul the contract incorporating Baylor University School of Medicine into the Southwestern Medical Foundation. It also publicly announced that Baylor University had received an offer from the M.D. Anderson Foundation (founded in Houston in 1936 by another wealthy Texan, Monroe D. Anderson, with much the same stated purpose as the Southwest Medical Foundation) to move the medical school from Dallas to Houston. Baylor University President Pat Neff told reporters "... the removal of the school of medicine at Dallas was caused by a breaking, on the part of the medical foundation, of the agreement.... 'The

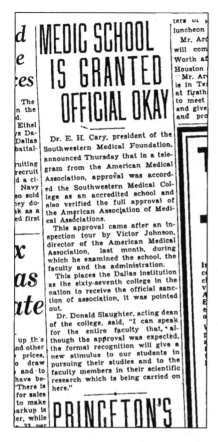

MEDIC SCHOOL IS GRANTED OFFICIAL OKAY

Dr. E. H. Cary, president of the Southwestern Medical Foundation, announced Thursday that in a telegram from the American Medical Association, approval was accorded the Southwestern Medical College as an accredited school and also verified the full approval of the American Association of Medical Associations.

This approval came after an inspection tour by Victor Johnson, director of the American Medical Association, last month, during which he examined the school, the faculty and the administration.

This places the Dallas institution as the sixty-seventh college in the nation to receive the official sanction of association, it was pointed out.

Dr. Donald Slaughter, acting dean of the college, said, "I can speak for the entire faculty that, although the approval was expected, the formal recognition will give a new stimulus to our students in pursuing their studies and to the faculty members in their scientific research which is being carried on here."

PRINCETON'S

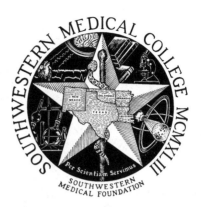

(Above) The seal of the Southwestern Medical College of the Southwestern Medical Foundation, established in 1943.

(Left) A Dallas newspaper announced the accreditation of the newly formed Southwestern Medical College by the American Medical Association.

trustees did not break the contract,' he said, declaring that 'Baptists do not break contracts.'"[7] Cary immediately responded. "Since Baylor had broken its contract, the Southwestern Medical Foundation would set up its own medical school in Dallas and do for it what had been planned for Baylor."[2] So the foundation "suddenly became the proprietor of part of a faculty and a sizable student body of a medical school."[6] Cary sought and received accreditation for the new school from the AMA and the American Association of Medical Associations. Such was the (inauspicious) beginning of the Southwestern Medical College of the Southwestern Medical Foundation.

The parting from Baylor University was hardly amicable. Not surprisingly, different accounts promote different sides of the story. According to John Chapman, Neff visited Dallas to invite the in-house medical students and the faculty to the new school in Houston. Most declined. When asked whether the new Southwestern Medical College would have access to the premises of the former Baylor University Medical College (for which there were no immediate plans), Neff declared, "'Under no circumstances.'... Workmen in the Baylor buildings were almost at that moment dismantling and preparing to ship to Houston everything salvable."[6] Walter Moursund, a former dean of the Baylor College of Medicine, provided a different account of events in his book, *History of Baylor University College of Medicine.*

> Many things were done to embarrass the Baylor Medical College. Pressure was brought to bear upon the salaried faculty to join the [Southwestern Medical] foundation school. Even the applicants who had been accepted for admission in the freshman class for the next year were besieged by telephone, telegraph, and other means to try to persuade them to accept admission to the new school. Attempts to embarrass the college were directed towards creating unfriendliness and non-cooperation among the members of the Houston medical profession. Since time has already written the history of both schools, the writer has no desire to record any more of the unfortunate events of the period of confusion.[13]

Notwithstanding the crisis situation, biographer Mooney's record of that time suggests a distinctly celebratory tone in Dallas—just cause for touting Cary's achievements. "One time there had been a young doctor fresh from New York, trying to get an apparently ill-starred medical school on its feet. Now there was an elder statesman of American medicine finding that the leaders of the city he adopted so many years before were eager and anxious to be of assistance."[2] Cary announced a bold fundraising campaign aimed at generating $1.5 million for the new medical school. One million was to be for new buildings, the rest for operations. "'Outstanding scientists and medical educators must be assured of a permanent, growing institution in this area,' Cary said. 'Research programs must be developed further by the addition of unusually able men to the faculty ... men who will be selected for their abilities both in research and teaching.'"[2] By November 1953, more than $1.3 million had been raised from individual contributions. Additionally, the Hoblitzelle Foundation, founded by theater magnate Karl Hoblitzelle, donated the amount required to purchase the land on Harry Hines Boulevard where the new medical school would be located.

"No man anywhere could have been happier than Cary on May 30, 1943, when ground was broken, an official spade being wielded by Mayor Woodall Rodgers," Booth Mooney wrote.[2] A Founders Day Dinner attended by 500 prominent Dallas citizens featured Cary as toastmaster and Dr. Chauncey Leake from the University of Texas Medical Branch at Galveston as the principal speaker. Leake was inspirational. "'If you are going to have a medical school, make it the

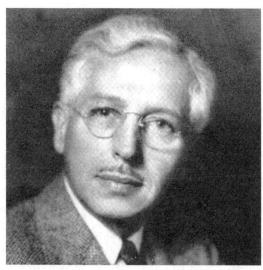

Often regarded more as a poet and philosopher than a theater magnate and banker, Karl Hoblitzelle made his fortune through his various business interests and created a legend through his philanthropy. In his partnership and friendship with Dr. E. H. Cary, Mr. Hoblitzelle provided much of the original financial base of Southwestern Medical Foundation, through the Hoblitzelle Foundation that he and his wife Esther created in 1942. The Foundation provided the funds that purchased 68 acres on Harry Hines Boulevard for the fledgling medical center.

greatest in the nation,' he implored. 'Let it be not only for the Southwest, but for the entire country. Let your horizons be as broad as they can be possibly be.'"[2]

The Southwestern Medical Foundation quickly obtained permission from the City of Dallas to occupy the empty (and dilapidated) Alex W. Spence Junior High School for a three-month period, and medical teaching continued. In May 1943, the final class of the original Baylor University College of Medicine graduated at a ceremony held at Southern Methodist University. In October of that year, the new medical school moved to the prefabricated army style barracks at 2211 Oak Lawn Avenue—where it would be housed for much longer than it hoped.

Meanwhile, Baylor University College of Medicine reopened in Houston, retaining its affiliation with Baylor University until 1969, when it became independent and changed its name to Baylor College of Medicine. That same year, the Texas legislature passed a bill that entitled the college to receive state tax dollars for providing medical education to Texas residents at the same rate as the state schools in Galveston and Dallas, while retaining its private status. Baylor College of Medicine is presently a thriving academic institution with

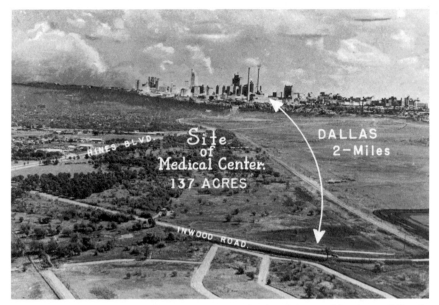

The original site for the Southwestern Medical School donated by the Hoblitzelle Foundation.

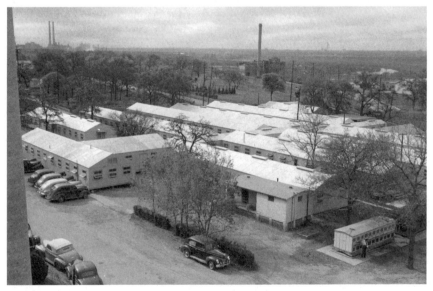

The Southwestern Medical College of the Southwest Medical Foundation was initially housed in prefabricated plywood army barracks located on Oak Lawn Avenue, close to the second Parkland Hospital.

an outstanding reputation in medical education and research and is a most worthy "local" academic rival of UT Southwestern. As a final note, the hospital that served the original Baylor University College of Medicine during its years in Dallas became a private non-university-affiliated hospital called Baylor University Medical Center. It endures to this day.

CHAPTER 4

THE UNIVERSITY OF TEXAS
SOUTHWESTERN MEDICAL
SCHOOL

Despite the enthusiastic rhetoric, the Southwestern Medical Foundation faced countless difficulties with its new orphan. The decrepit Alex Spence School was only tenable as an emergency facility. Moreover, it was wartime—building supplies and manpower were in short supply, and rationing was the order of the day. "Hardware and plumbing supplies were almost unobtainable, and if bits and pieces did turn up, it was next to impossible to find a mechanic who knew how to put them together."[1] The school had to be accredited, salaries had to be secured for the seventeen remaining faculty, and 277 admissions applications had arrived. Finally, and perhaps most importantly, the dissolution from Baylor University meant that the medical school in Dallas was once again without university affiliation.

The Dallas-based Eighth Service Command of the U.S. Army authorized the construction of 30,000 square feet of prefabricated barracks on Oak Lawn Avenue and provided salaries, tuition, and fees. After all, the school provided a potential source of much-needed doctors, and most of the students were in military service on detached duty. While the architecture was no more stylish than "henhouse classic,"[1] the "shacks" were functional and convenient to Parkland Hospital (then also located on Oak Lawn Avenue). Dr. Donald Slaughter was appointed acting dean. The full-time faculty included only nine individuals, all appointed to teach basic sciences. The remaining faculty consisted of practicing clinicians who worked part-time for the medical school, for which they were paid modest honoraria.

✳ ✳ ✳ ✳ ✳

In addition to securing a temporary home, albeit one in which neither the walls nor the floor were more than three quarters of an inch thick, the medical school added several distinguished individuals to its full-time faculty in

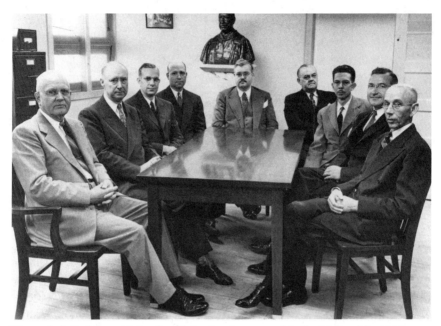

The only full-time paid faculty of the Southwestern Medical School in 1943 were professors in the basic science departments. They were (from left to right) Charles Duncan, histology; George Caldwell, pathology; Joseph T. Hill, clinical pathology; Robert Lackey, physiology; Don Slaughter, pharmacology (Dr. Slaughter also functioned as acting dean of the school); Lewis Waters (medical art, not a faculty member); Herbert Tidwall, biochemistry; MacDonald Fulton, microbiology; and William Looney, anatomy.

its first year of operation. The highly regarded cardiologist and innovator in medical education, Tinsley R. Harrison (then at Vanderbilt University), was appointed chairman of the Department of Internal Medicine; the brilliant academic surgeon Carl Moyer was appointed professor of Experimental Surgery in the Department of Surgery; and Arthur Grollman, a nationally recognized physiologist and an authority on hypertension (with MD and PhD degrees from Johns Hopkins), served simultaneously as chairman of the Department of Physiology and the Department of Pharmacology.

While at Southwestern Medical College, Harrison wrote his famous medical textbook, *Principles of Internal Medicine.* This text, used by generations of students throughout the world, entered its 15th edition in 2001, and at the time of this writing had sold close to three million copies! When sales surpassed one million, Jean Wilson, a distinguished faculty member in the Department of Internal Medicine at UT Southwestern and one of the book's ed-

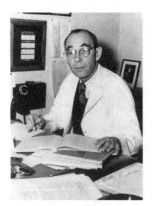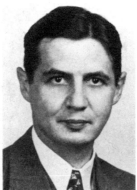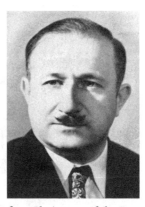

(Left) Tinsley Randolph Harrison (1900–1978) was the first Chairman of the Department of Internal Medicine at Southwestern Medical School. Harrison edited the first five editions of *Harrison's Principles of Internal Medicine*, a renowned textbook used worldwide. Harrison used the box shown above the telephone to communicate with his secretary in the adjacent office. He served as dean of the school from 1944–1946.

(Center) Carl Alfred Moyer (1908–1970), a highly regarded experimental surgeon, served as Dean of Southwestern Medical School during 1950–1951 and later chaired the Department of Surgery at the University of Washington, St. Louis.

(Right) Arthur Grollman (1901–1980). After acquiring the MD and PhD degrees at Johns Hopkins, Grollman was a professor at several schools around the nation before moving to Dallas in 1947 to become Professor of Medicine and Chairman of the Departments of Physiology and Pharmacology at Southwestern Medical School.

itors, authored a monograph on its history. On the 100th anniversary of Harrison's birth, Wilson presented part of this history at the University of Alabama in Birmingham, where Harrison spent his remaining academic career after leaving Southwestern in 1950. "Harrison's *Principles of Internal Medicine* was founded at Southwestern Medical College and a large number of the authors of the first edition were from Dallas,"[2] Wilson related. "In addition to Harrison himself, who also served as editor-in-chief, chapters were contributed by John Chapman, Gladys Fashena, Ben Friedman, Mort Mason, Carl Moyer, Andrew Small, Elias Strauss and Paul Williams. Prior to Harrison, textbooks of medicine were very empirical. His was the first book to integrate clinical medicine and pathophysiology—and it had a huge impact."[2]

Harrison was not the foundation's first choice for the chairmanship of the Department of Internal Medicine. Irvine McQuarrie, chairman of the Pedi-

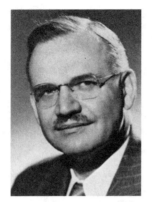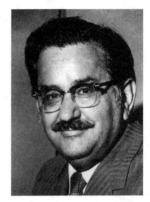

(Left) William F. Mengert, Chairman of the Department of Obstetrics and Gynecology at Southwestern Medical School, worked at the University of Iowa School of Medicine with the renowned obstetrician E. D. Plass. Mengert served as acting dean at Southwestern in 1946.

(Right) Simon Edward Sulkin (1908–1972) was the second—but the first major—Chairman of the Department of Microbiology, from 1945–1972. Dr. Sulkin was noted for his pioneering studies on the natural history of rabies virus infection. His widow, Ms. Lorraine Sulkin Schein, established three separate endowments honoring the visionary work, standard of scientific excellence, and memory of Dr. Sulkin.

atrics Department at the University of Minnesota Medical School, was offered the position first and turned it down. But "Harrison had a dramatic impact as a speaker at the annual meeting of the Texas Medical Association [in 1943]. Among the impressed audience were some Dallas internists who proposed him as a candidate for the chairmanship of internal medicine to Cary."[2] This recommendation was accepted and Harrison's appointment was formalized in March 1944. A condition of his appointment, to which he reluctantly agreed, was that he also serve as dean of the medical school. Harrison "did not like being dean.... [H]e was not successful at raising money in the community and did not work well with the executive director of the [Southwestern Medical] Foundation. The Board thought he spent too much money and he resigned the post after two years."[2]

As dean, Harrison recruited both Grollman and Moyer to the Southwestern faculty. He also recruited William Mengert, a prominent figure in obstetrics and gynecology; S. Edward Sulkin, one of the early "microbe hunters" during the Golden Age of Microbiology (noted for his pioneering studies on the natural history of rabies virus infection); and the pediatrician Gilbert Forbes, for whom Forbes' disease (a hereditary deficiency characterized by the

storage of short chain glycogen molecules) is named, and who made important contributions to understanding the influence of androgens on body mass.
"The net consequence of these various appointments was to give the young
medical school instant credibility."[2] Given that the school's budget was a mere
$200,000, these appointments were substantial achievements. During the dif-
ficult war years, Harrison also maintained an active investigative program and
attracted medical students to his research laboratory.

As the war drew to a close, the spirit at the medical school was enthusiastic. Dr. Gladys Fashena, from the Department of Pediatrics, commented, "she
had never been associated with a medical school in which the morale was so
high.... In part it seems to have been the kind of attitude that develops in a
group engaged in a difficult undertaking of any sort. In part the morale seems
to have been generated by the personalities of the full-time faculty. Certainly
Harrison contributed a very considerable share."[1]

This indefatigable confidence and pride in the school and its achievements
endures. Though now secure in its reputation as one of the premier academic
medical centers in the world, recruiting distinguished faculty to UT Southwestern remains a challenge, and distinguished faculty recruitments continue
to be celebrated as triumphs. Located near the southern border of the great
plains, the city's surroundings are monotonously flat. Summers are grim, and,
as already mentioned, Dallas remains best known in the minds of many as the
site of the Kennedy assassination. Many privately (and some even publicly)
avow that for too long, Dallas's only notable cultural features were the TV
show of the same name and the football team, the Dallas Cowboys. But in
fact, one has to live in the city to understand that while the summers are indeed hot, the rest of the year is climatically delightful. Moreover, the city is
home to a world-class opera company and symphony orchestra. Together with
its twin city, Fort Worth, it hosts some of the finest art museums in the world
and its restaurants can satisfy the most discerning palate.

※ ※ ※ ※ ※

With the medical school off to a promising start in the mid-1940s, what
prompted Harrison, Moyer, and others to leave? Jean Wilson explained.

> For one thing, the school fell on hard times financially. The only sup-
> port was from the Southwestern Medical Foundation. The assump-
> tion that the school would be able to raise philanthropic money did
> not materialize—at least not at that time. So there was a severe fi-
> nancial crisis. The only solution was to be rescued by the state. Then
> too, perhaps in part as a result of the financial problems, these dis-

tinguished chairmen were being offered positions elsewhere. Moyer went to a prestigious appointment at Washington University in St. Louis, Forbes went to Rochester (New York), and Mengert went to the University of Illinois. All these places were more established and had bigger budgets and departments than we did at Southwestern.[2]

It was Harrison's departure, however, that prompted the others to leave. "Harrison's departure is something of a mystery," Wilson stated. "His public excuse was that he feared take over of the school by the State of Texas; that the state rather than the faculty would control the curriculum. But this made little sense because he left Southwestern for another state school, a new medical school being built in Birmingham, Alabama."[2]

Others have commented on Harrison's alleged concern about state control of the medical school. Biographer James Pittman of the University of Alabama notes: "Soon after Harrison learned that Southwestern would probably become a branch of the University of Texas with a [considerably expanded] entering class of one hundred, he submitted his resignation, stating as his reason that classes of one hundred were simply too large."[3] But personal problems also complicated Harrison's sojourn in Dallas. "He never neglected a student, and only rarely his research; but perhaps he took his family for granted. His wife Betty must have felt alone ... and in 1949 ... she proposed to move back to Nashville, where they had probably been happiest, and he talked of returning to private practice."[3]

⁂ ⁂ ⁂ ⁂ ⁂

Notwithstanding the fundraising campaign orchestrated by the Southwestern Medical Foundation and the acquisition of land on Harry Hines Boulevard, by 1947 construction on the new medical school still had not commenced. "Not even the stroke of a hammer was audible."[1] The complexities of local and state politics, coupled with post-war shortages of supplies and labor left the school languishing in the shacks. Cary became increasingly convinced that "the future of the school demanded far more adequate support than the [Southwestern Medical] Foundation would be able to provide, at least for some years to come."[1] Furthermore, while plans to gain university affiliation for Southwestern Medical College had been in the forefront of Cary's mind since the school's inception in 1943, none of the geographically obvious institutions were attractive. "Private schools in the area, the strongest of which were Texas Christian University in Fort Worth and Southern Methodist University in Dallas, could barely meet their budgets. [Besides], the past experiences with Baylor peremptorily excluded consideration of affiliation with any denominational university.... There remained a [single] remote, but not impossible, alliance—one with the University of Texas,"[1] two hundred miles to the south in Austin, but already with a Medical School Branch in Galveston.

"Cary began quiet and private discussions with Dudley K. Woodward, an accessible acquaintance, a lawyer, and a gentleman from Dallas who happened at that time to be chairman of the Board of Regents of the University of Texas. Naturally there are no records of these conversations, but it would be quite inconceivable that the medical school at Dallas was not a subject of occasional discussion."[1] Eventually, the way was paved for the state legislature to pass a bill establishing a second medical school in the University of Texas System, the location of which was to be determined by the House of Delegates of the Texas Medical Association.

When the University of Texas System invited formal applications these were received from San Antonio, El Paso, Temple, and Dallas. "The vote of the House of Delegates [of the Texas Medical Association] was seventy-nine to fifty-four in favor of Dallas [and] Dr. Cary is reported to have poured himself a double bourbon and retired to a most peaceful sleep that night."[1] In 1949, the Southwestern Medical Foundation gifted the Southwestern Medical College to the state, and the school became officially known as the Southwestern Medical School of the University of Texas.

Initially, Southwestern Medical School was established as a statutory branch of the university, not a constitutional branch like the school in Galveston. In this capacity it did not qualify for allocations directly from the university's permanent fund; instead, it had to appeal annually to the state legislature for its operational support and construction funds (until a constitutional amendment was adopted years later). The Texas legislature was not particularly forthcoming with financial appropriations, especially for major construction costs. John Chapman notes, "Dallas's fight to make the University of Texas a gift of Southwestern Medical School had won few friends [elsewhere in the state] and influenced a good many people unfavorably. Having adopted the orphan medical school, the state apparently was not of a mind to spoil it. The delegation from San Antonio in particular had taken offense … and Dean Carl Moyer received rough treatment as he presented the proposed budget in February, 1951"[1] (although the legislature ultimately appropriated $2.75 million in 1951 to erect the first permanent building). So the celebrations that attended the opening of the 1950–51 academic year notwithstanding, many considered the Southwestern Medical School to be "in very sad disarray."[1]

With Harrison's departure, the young and relatively inexperienced dean of the medical school, Carl Moyer, was recruited to Washington University in St. Louis, where he became one of the great experimental surgeons of his generation and co-authored another celebrated textbook, *Surgery: Principles and Practice*. The additional loss of Charles Burnett, Harrison's successor to the chair of the Department of Internal Medicine, after less than a year in Dallas left the acting chairmanship in the hands of neurologist Tom Farmer. He too departed soon after, to join Burnett in North Carolina. "Perhaps neither Moyer nor Burnett had been prepared for the labyrinthine channels of the University of Texas, or the activities of rural politicians, who at that time dominated the legislature."[1] This was the somewhat desperate academic and financial environment that faced the thirty-one-year-old Donald Seldin when he arrived in Dallas early in 1951.

CHAPTER 5

THE EARLY SELDIN YEARS

Born in Coney Island on October 24, 1920, Donald (Don) Wayne Seldin was the son of Jewish parents who fled persecution in Eastern Europe at the end of the 19th century. His dentist father was a scholarly man, fluent in Hebrew, Latin, and Greek, but Seldin claims that little of this scholarship rubbed off on him. "I was enrolled in Hebrew School, [but] I never attended classes. My own interest was to distinguish myself in a gang and play football and baseball."[1] Tall and rangy, Seldin played basketball on a championship James Madison High School team in New York City, and ran the 100-yard dash on the track team. But his macho protestations notwithstanding, Seldin's home environment clearly did influence his intellectual development—during his high school years he cultivated wide-ranging scholarly interests including literature, poetry, and political science.[1]

When the Great Depression forced Seldin's father into bankruptcy he turned to the business world to supplement his dental practice—an experience that prompted his conviction that in order to succeed financially one had to be a business man, not a professional. So when Seldin decided to apply to medical school his father was decidedly unsupportive. And when years later he announced that he would be joining the faculty of a relatively unknown medical school in Dallas, Texas (of all places) rather than entering private practice in New York, an established bastion of culture and success, his father considered the move nothing short of disastrous.

Seldin entered Yale Medical School in 1943, the year that the Southwest Medical Foundation launched its unknown medical college. Yale then boasted a distinguished Department of Internal Medicine headed by Francis Blake, a capable leader who oversaw the department's twenty-year transformation from a single salaried professor and a few part-time faculty in the early 1920s to a highly respected academic department.[2] A superb clinician with a broad knowledge of medicine and astute diagnostic abilities, Blake was nationally recognized for his research on epidemic diseases and directed some of the first clinical tests on penicillin and sulfonamide drugs. He strongly encouraged his faculty colleagues to augment their clinical responsibilities with teaching and

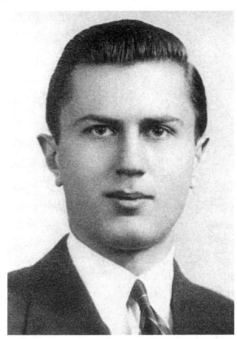

Donald Wayne Seldin, often referred to as "the grandfather of UT Southwestern," as a medical student at Yale University. At the time of this writing Seldin holds the William Buchanan Chair in Internal Medicine and a University of Texas System Professorship in Internal Medicine. He is a member of the Institute of Medicine of the U.S. National Academy of Sciences, and was awarded the prestigious Kobler Medal from the Association of American Physicians in 1985.

research, and Seldin refers to Blake as the epitome of the clinical scholar, a term coined to describe physicians with serious academic aspirations. "He sponsored academic work and research such that the metabolic division [in the Department of Internal Medicine] became the rallying point for anyone interested in academic medicine and research at Yale Medical School."[1]

Blake brought with him to Yale a brilliant clinical investigator and outspoken nonconformist, John Punnett Peters. Peters conducted extensive research, writing books and articles at a fierce pace. His 1932 reference book, *Quantitative Clinical Chemistry* (written with Donald D. Van Slyke), had an enormous impact on clinical research and medical practice around the world. Peters urged residents to ground their care of patients in scientific principles and he "supervised a large coterie of research fellows," many of who went on to distinguished academic careers.[2] Peters was noted for his work in metabolism and created an outstanding academically-focused renal center at the Grace-

New Haven Community Hospital. "I was deeply impressed by his learning, scholarship and dedication to medicine, all integrated together,"[1] Seldin said. Both Blake and Peters were powerful role models for Seldin, influencing his unwavering commitment to academic medicine.

* * * * *

Like many of his classmates and peers around the country, Seldin enlisted in the U.S. Army while in medical school. In 1946, following his internship and residency training at Yale, he was activated for military service and dispatched to the 98th General Hospital in Munich, Germany, where he remained for two years. Seldin served as the chief of a sizable medical service and established and operated a state-of-the-art clinical laboratory at the hospital—all at the age of twenty-six.

Seldin's many colleagues and adversaries will attest not only to his outstanding administrative and organizational talents, but to his unbending will, his single-mindedness, and his strength of character. As a young army captain in Germany, he testified as an expert witness in the military trial of a

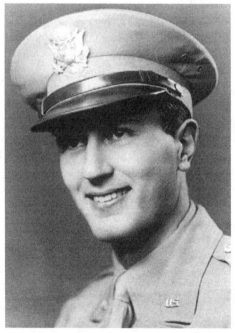

Don Seldin enlisted in the U.S. Army Medical Corps during World War II and served at the 98th General Hospital in Munich, Germany.

Nazi physician accused of causing the deaths of some forty patients by need-lessly performing liver biopsies when they were in the active phase of hepa-titis. Seldin's account of that experience captures the essence of his forceful personality:

> The trial had been going on for some time before I was asked to tes-tify. The general officers serving as judges decided that if the liver biopsies had been done with a therapeutic intent, the deaths, how-ever tragic, would not be considered murder. But if the biopsies were done without informed consent for experimental purposes, or for torture, the physician would be convicted of murder. The question I was summoned to answer essentially was, what was the place of liver biopsy at that time? I was asked [to testify] ... because at that time I was probably one of the few senior medical officers remaining in Eu-rope following the return of many to the U.S. at the end of the war.
>
> The accused German physician was very smart and was acting as his own attorney. He was fluent in English and had had fellowship training at the Rockefeller Institute before the war. When he exam-ined me, his first approach was to challenge my competence by quizzing me extensively on methods for measuring liver function. [His approach was that] if one was an expert witness on liver biopsy one ought to know about liver tests. He had the Peters and Van Slyke textbook in front of him and he asked me, 'How do you fractionate the serum proteins?' 'How do you do this?' 'How do you do that?' For-tuitously, these were things that I had at my fingertips. I had learned them at Yale in Peters' laboratory, and I had just set up the clinical laboratory in Munich. So I had no trouble answering his questions. We went back and forth on this and I kept pointing out that what-ever the purpose of liver biopsy, it couldn't be used to direct therapy. Finally, the court decided that this was not a procedure done remotely in the interests of the patients. Forty patients dying following liver biopsy pointed to medical inhumanity, not medical therapy. [The German physician] was convicted and sentenced.[1]

When the time came to return to the United States, Seldin was undecided about his professional future. But on his last day in Germany he providentially received a letter from his former mentor at Yale, John Peters. "Dear Don," the terse note read. "I would like to offer you a position as Instructor of Medicine at a salary beginning at $2,500 a year. Why haven't you written? Sincerely yours, Jack."[3] Seldin accepted the offer without batting an eyelid, and within a year he was promoted to the rank of Assistant Professor of Medicine at Yale.

With more than a half dozen publications to his credit, Seldin was well on his way to a promising academic career.

✻ ✻ ✻ ✻ ✻

Following Harrison's abrupt departure from Southwestern Medical School a search committee identified Charles (Chuck) Burnett as the new chairman of the Department of Internal Medicine. Burnett was a former student of the famous Harvard endocrinologist Fuller Albright, considered the founder of the study of metabolic bone diseases and the father of modern endocrinology. Burnett is immortalized in the annals of academic medicine from his description of the clinical syndrome that bears his name, a clinical entity caused by long-term calcium and alkali ingestion.

Sometime in 1950 Don Seldin received an unexpected phone call from Burnett, whom he had never met. "He called me to ask if I might be interested in setting up an academic program in the medical service that he was going to develop in Dallas." [3] Seldin related. There were many reasons why Seldin might not have entertained such an offer. "My wife Muriel and I really loved the northeast—and I didn't know or care anything at all about Texas. Muriel had lived in New York and Long Island all her life. In addition, Yale provided a highly stimulating environment independent of my career in academic medicine. Muriel loved music and participated in the Yale music school when the famous composer Paul Hindemith was dean. And we knew and socialized with a lot of interesting people there. All in all we had a very complete and satisfying life in New Haven, with no particular desire to leave."[3]

Years later, when on the other side of the recruiting table as a department chair, Seldin came to fully appreciate the complex dynamics of acquiring talented faculty. "I quickly learned that when one wants to recruit someone to a new position in academia it's extremely helpful if in addition to the 'pull' of what one is offering to someone, there are also factors pushing them to leave where they are. If for some reason, be it personal, social, political or academic, an individual is dissatisfied with what he or she has, it's easier for them to seriously examine an attractive offer. But in my case the reality then was that I wasn't being pushed in any way. Peters wanted me to stay at Yale—and I was very happy there."[3] Nonetheless, Seldin admits that in retrospect he can identify several aspects of life at Yale University that helped "push" him to Dallas. For one thing, notwithstanding his promising beginnings as a young faculty member, he recognized that there was precious little room at the top of the academic ladder in the Yale Department of Internal Medicine.

The Department of Internal Medicine at Yale was very crowded in the area in which I was working—metabolic studies. If I stayed at Yale I would be fifth or sixth—or even later in line behind a group of first-rate people who were senior to me. Additionally, developing an independent research program at Yale wasn't that easy. Peters didn't allow any technicians in the research labs and so you had to do your own experimental work. It was also difficult to carry out many types of metabolic studies because there were no metabolic wards at Yale. And Peters himself almost never did experimental work on animals, so there wasn't any established animal research either.[1]

Seldin also didn't particularly mind leaving some of the subtle but disturbing social influences he'd experienced at Yale.

I'm sure that there was some concern about the fact that I was Jewish. Peters later told me that when I graduated from medical school in 1943 at the top of my class the President of Yale, Charles Seymour, called him and said: 'Doctor, I understand one of your students is getting the Campbell Gold Medal [the highest honor in the graduating class].' Dr. Peters replied, 'Yes.' Dr. Seymour said, 'I assume the recipient, Mr. Seldin, comes from a family that has attended Yale for many years.' 'No he does not,' Peters responded. 'Well then, I assume then that they went to other schools like Harvard or Dartmouth.' Peters said 'No,' again. 'Well, probably the family has been in this country for many years, many generations.' Peters said, 'No.' After this, there was a pause and Peters said, 'Look, I should tell you that his parents are immigrants. They never went to college here. He is the first member of his family to be in an American university.'[1]

But most overwhelmingly, Seldin was a natural academic leader; a physician-scholar brimming with ambition and enthusiasm, and he was fundamentally intrigued by the long-term prospects of Burnett's offer. Here was an opportunity to build his own academic unit, albeit in a little known medical school in a part of the country about which he knew nothing. Indeed, the more he thought about it the more he saw the relative obscurity of Southwestern as an opportunity rather than a deterrent.

Opportunities to have your own academic unit didn't come around all that often, especially in those days. After all, there weren't that many academically oriented medical schools in the country at that time. The thing in Dallas was one of the more minor developments going on in the country. But I thought that it might be exciting. I decided that I shouldn't and couldn't turn down an opportunity to build something on my own. Besides, I was young and I realized that I didn't have to be in Dallas forever. So I decided to accept Burnett's offer. I took the job, sight unseen. I never came to Dallas to see the place. It sounds unbelievable, but in those days money wasn't available for that sort of traveling. People didn't readily fly young assistant professors around the country and wine and dine them as we do today.[3]

But immediately following his arrival in Dallas Seldin found precious little to reinforce his enthusiasm. Construction of the proposed new medical school showed no signs of materializing, the plans for a new Parkland Hospital were languishing, and the already thin faculty was becoming thinner.

It was not at all clear when, if ever, we would ever get a new hospital—or even a new medical school. And with Burnett's departure things were really in a bad state. There was almost no full-time faculty in the Department of Internal Medicine. Even the part-time faculty was far too thin and there was essentially no leadership. In fact the school was on probation with respect to its accreditation. In addition, there was a lot of tension in the physician community about its relationship to the medical school; tensions about whether people should be allowed to have private patients—and that sort of thing. The relationship with Parkland Hospital was also in an awkward state. For example, John Goode was chairman of the Department of Surgery in the medical school, but he wasn't chief of the Parkland Hospital surgical service and this sort of arrangement generated obvious tensions.[3]

Seldin's description of the shacks he found in January 1951 was no exaggeration. As John Chapman incisively commented: "Southwestern in the fall of 1952 was probably appealing only to academic types with a considerable spirit of adventure. In 1948 a fire in the area of [Tinsley] Harrison's laboratory and office had left ineradicable traces.... Here and there water leaks had led to softening of the bonding that held together thin lamellae of plywood, with the result that now and again a heavy piece of laboratory instrument or even a chair leg would go through the floor. Since the buildings had no formal foundation, they leaned rather informally away from the prevailing winds. In one place or another one could see the rich earth of Texas between walls and floor. When the wind was strong that same rich earth made its way into the buildings."[4]

Nor was Parkland Hospital in much better shape. "A candidate for the professorship in medicine, having toured the medical wards, remarked that though he had served in hospitals in New York and other eastern cities, he had never seen anything as rough. He added rather acidly that he would not care to teach in a city that permitted patients to be hospitalized under such conditions."[4] When neurologist Tom Farmer decided to accompany Burnett to the University of North Carolina, Seldin was the sole remaining full-time faculty member in the Department of Medicine!

For all of his ambition and resolve, this situation gave Seldin considerable pause, especially since as word of the potential collapse of the medical school circulated through the academic grapevine, offers surfaced to move the talented young clinical scholar to less troubled waters.

> I had an offer to go with Burnett to North Carolina. I also had an offer to return to Yale, and there was a tentative offer in the works to go to Harvard. For a while things were really up in the air. Muriel and I had not yet purchased a house in Dallas. We had a rented apartment. But after Burnett and Farmer left we gave the apartment up and Muriel went back to New Haven to look for a place for us to live in. I stayed with Sam Shelbourne, a practitioner in town and a friend of mine. For a while it looked as if we really would be returning to New Haven. But several things developed that seemed promising to me. One was that I was told by several reputable sources that Governor Allan Shivers was committed to putting up a new building for the medical school. Second, the Commissioner's Court of Dallas County announced that it would launch a bond issue for a new Parkland Hospital adjacent to the new medical school building.[3]

Buoyed by the prospect of imminent relief and a rosier future, Seldin decided to wait and see. Also on the plus side was the reality that though still modest in size and scope, his research program was slowly beginning to unfold with pleasing prospects. "A number of medical students were already working in my laboratory on various projects. They were absolutely outstanding and the work was going well. And last but by no means least, when George Aagaard was interviewed for the deanship of the medical school I liked what I heard him say about developing academic programs here."[3] After all was said and done, Seldin, like Cary, was fundamentally reluctant to forgo his vision. While many considered Southwestern Medical School an embryonic lower tier institution unlikely to rise to national prominence, Seldin viewed the school as an unspoiled opportunity, a place not yet molded by established tradition and biases, a place where he could realize his aspirations of clinical scholarship. He was already convinced that Dallas had no shortage of bright and motivated students, and, like Cary, he genuinely appreciated the Texan friendliness and can-do mentality. Ultimately, he decided to remain at Southwestern—at least for the moment.

Following Harrison's brief term as dean, the medical school was successively served in this capacity by William Lee Hart (1946–50) and Carl Moyer (1950–51). In 1952, George Aagaard, an experienced administrator from the University of Minnesota Medical School, was appointed to the position. Aagaard had his work cut out for him. First, he had to fill the glaring vacancies in departmental chairmanships. Second, he had to push on with the building program. Then followed innumerable lesser problems. Quick to recognize the potential of the bright and aggressive young man from Yale, Aagaard designated Seldin as acting chairman of the Department of Internal Medicine. A year later he removed the temporary nature of this appointment. In a mere two years Seldin was elevated from Instructor of Medicine at Yale University to Professor and Chairman of the Department of Internal Medicine at Southwestern Medical School. At the age of thirty-two he was actively recruiting faculty, building a comprehensive clinical service, establishing a credible resi-

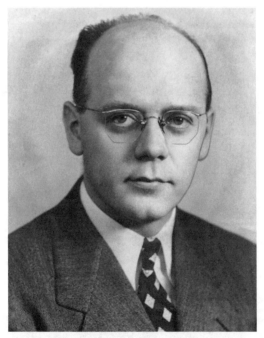

George Aagaard served as dean of the University of Texas Southwestern Medical School from 1952–1954, before departing to a highly successful tenure as dean of the School of Medicine at the University of Washington.

dency training program, and introducing state-of-the-art clinical research. The Dallas medical school was once again on the move.

In the early 1950s, Texas Governor Allan Shivers (who is credited by many for setting the stage for the emergence of Texas as a powerful modern state) led a delegation from Austin to Dallas to determine whether the legislature should appropriate funds for the construction of permanent buildings at Southwestern Medical College. The visit strongly reinforced how badly the medical school needed help. Philip O'Bryan (P.O.B.) Montgomery, Jr., a former faculty member in the Department of Pathology and later a special assistant to the president's office at UT Southwestern, relates: "Students, fellows and faculty were lined up in the shacks to welcome the governor and his entourage. The governor entered through the back of one of the long shacks and when he had walked half way through this edifice a window simply dropped out of the wall. The governor continued walking, and about a hundred feet further one of his feet went through the floor. We knew from the look on his face that he was going to help us."[4]

At Yale, Seldin inherited a philosophy from his mentors that he never abandoned—that the practice of medicine and the pursuit of knowledge in the med-

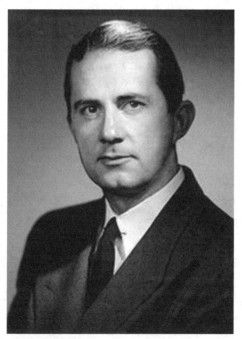

Robert Allan Shivers (1907–1985) served as Governor of Texas for three terms from 1949–1957. He visited Southwestern Medical School in the early 1950s.

ical and basic sciences must progress simultaneously. He elaborated on this philosophy at length one morning in his office, a room crowded with papers, books,
journals and other assorted bric-a-brac. (His assistant informed me that some
of this material had occupied the floor of Seldin's office since he first arrived fifty
years ago!) He eagerly discussed his views on the role of the clinician-scientist
in academic medicine, ideas well encapsulated in his 1966 Presidential Address
to the *58th Annual Meeting of the American Society for Clinical Investigation.*

> Research in a medical school subserves two functions. Investigation is
> by definition the search for truth, the discovery of new knowledge, the
> development of explanatory and predictive theories. [But] if this were
> all, a University would be no different from a research institute. Clearly
> the University has the vital additional function of education.... Only the
> investigator can inculcate the methods of critical inquiry acquired in re-
> search into the routine practice of medicine. Only he can bring physi-
> ology and biochemistry meaningfully to bear in the study and treatment
> of the sick. The practice of medicine, no matter how skillfully and re-
> sponsibly conducted, becomes progressively removed from the science
> of medicine to the extent that the clinician is no longer an investigator.[5]

Elsewhere Seldin stated, "[a]t the level of the medical student, it's very important that the medical school establish a culture of excitement about medicine and establish biomedical science as the basis of medicine. There are many
healers in society, but the only healer who brings medical *science* to the patient is the physician."[1]

Seldin's determination to emulate the clinical scholarship he had absorbed
at Yale in the embryonic facility at Southwestern Medical School is nothing
short of astonishing. One might even consider it naive. Certainly, some considered it foolish. "Peters didn't doubt that people would be medically responsible in Dallas," Seldin related. "He also thought there would be probably be a good teaching program there. But he couldn't believe that the place
would value my interest in research. He thought it would be virtually impossible for me to develop an academic program in Dallas, and he thought that
coming here was a very bad choice."[1]

Notwithstanding the frustrating local limitations, however, the general academic climate in biomedicine in the United States was ripe for such a bold
experiment. Seldin fortuitously brought his academic vision to Dallas at the
beginning of one the greatest revolutions in biology, a revolution that yielded
the structure of the gene and the unraveling of the genetic code, and that ushered in the era of a new discipline called molecular biology—a synthesis of genetics and biochemistry that promised untold dividends in comprehending

cellular function. The remainder of the twentieth century (and beyond) would witness spectacular progress in the biological sciences, and their integration into clinical medicine and the swift extension of molecular biology to molecular medicine would exceed even Seldin's wildest expectations.

By the middle of the twentieth century the United States had enormously strengthened research and educational funding through the National Institutes of Health (NIH). This vehicle of support for biomedical research, education, and specialized clinical care had its origins as early as 1930, when Joseph Randall, a Louisiana senator "dreamed of creating a great medical research institution in which hundreds of scholars would work on the underlying basis of all the diseases of humankind."[6] At the end of World War II, spurred on in part by the challenge to American technological superiority from the Russian space program, the NIH was greatly expanded, and by 1960 its annual appropriation reached $400 million. Some of these funds were, and still are, used to support the intramural (in-house) research program. But most was, as it is today, dedicated to the extramural program (outside research and education, mainly provided as grants to universities and colleges on the basis of competitive proposals). During the period of this considerable financial largesse, which extended into the 1980s, the majority of thoughtfully crafted proposals for biomedical research and training were favorably considered, a situation that is, regrettably, no longer the case. Seldin and his growing young faculty made extensive use of the opportunities afforded by NIH grants.

✻ ✻ ✻ ✻ ✻

Seldin lost little time in establishing and promoting his own research program at Southwestern, though not without considerable pleading and cajoling.

> Of course there was nothing in place. I had to purchase everything from scratch and I spent a great deal of time in a warehouse in downtown Dallas looking through catalogs. We had some money for minor pieces of equipment. But major pieces of equipment were not features of the laboratory at that time. About the most expensive item was a flame photometer. I also tried to develop a clinical research center at Parkland. I informed the hospital administrator that I needed four metabolic beds and a small kitchen so that we could prepare the special meals required for studies on patients with metabolic diseases. The hospital was very cooperative. In particular, even though this was a time before formal racial desegregation, the hospital administration was sufficiently forward looking that they allowed me to house patients of different ethnicity in this little four-bed ward.[3]

The new chairman of the Department of Internal Medicine also faced other contentious departmental issues head on. Though the department was seriously strapped for cash, many of the part-time faculty, who were physicians in private practice, were paid modest sums to teach medical students. Seldin adamantly reclaimed these fees. "In the end it amounted to a mere few thousand dollars, but there wasn't much money outside of that either, so I reclaimed it. Of course this caused a lot of fuss. The physicians who were paid to teach took pride in lecturing at the medical school and, even though the sums didn't amount to much, they were an important token of appreciation. But I felt that I needed that money for more important things."[3]

Amidst considerable protest from some members of the part-time clinical faculty, Seldin also revised the curriculum of lectures from top to bottom.

> There were a lot of lectures for students in their clinical training years, but they were not well organized. We had orthopedic lectures, surgical lectures, obstetrical lectures, pediatrics lectures, and medicine lectures, all in a period of time assigned to teaching clinical medicine in the broadest sense. I instituted a block system of teaching in which different subjects were taught in different blocks of time. In so doing I brought the teaching of medicine under the direct control of the Department of Internal Medicine. Additionally, instead of having the students subjected to lecture after lecture, sometimes all day long, with minor attendance on the wards, the emphasis was reversed. Students were required to concentrate mainly on their patients, and lectures were moved to a single afternoon a week. I also didn't think it appropriate to try to cover the vast topic of internal medicine exclusively through didactic lectures. This meant that some of the local practitioners were eliminated from the lecture program, either because I didn't think this or that person should present lectures, or because I thought that the subject matter was not appropriate. This too caused a tremendous fuss.[3]

Seldin was uncompromising in restructuring the curriculum of lectures and in introducing cutting edge academic medicine. The following example (one of many) typifies his resolve to modernize his department.

> I drastically reduced the number of lectures in dermatology because I felt that dermatology at that time was a primitive discipline in terms of solid scientific knowledge. Of course I immediately had a visit from a delegation of dermatologists. They argued that ninety percent of people who went to a physician had dermatologic problems. I had also added a lecture on porphyria (a disease popularized by the med-

ical history of King George III of England) and they wanted to know why I had done so when this was such a rare disease. I tried to convince them that the purpose of the porphyria lecture was not to teach the students about porphyria per se, but to give them a sense of how understanding a well known metabolic pathway can help elucidate a disease state. I would have to say that in those early days the faculty was quite upset by the changes, and by the many meetings called as a result—some of which were rather heated![3]

Seldin's knowledge of academic clinical medicine and his diagnostic acumen were legendary. Joe Goldstein (one of UT Southwestern's Nobel Laureates, about whom much more is told later) once described him as "the Toscanini of the student CPC [Clinico-Pathologic Conference]. If a patient with pernicious anemia was presented to Dr. Seldin, he would tell [you] the remarkable story of how William Castle discovered intrinsic factor.... To paraphrase the Seldin dictum of the 1960s,... each sick patient has a sick molecule and the route to medical progress is to investigate sick patients and their sick molecules."[7]

Seldin was never one to suffer fools lightly. An incorrect answer from a medical student is said to have prompted him to toss the hapless (and terrified) student a dime, with the acid retort, "Here's a dime. Go call your mother!" On more than one occasion he threw open a window on the Parkland wards and yelled, "Police! Police! Help! Someone is trying to kill my patient!"[1] In a nutshell, Seldin was a visible, charismatic and highly influential teacher to medical students, residents, and faculty. A colorful and energetic presence who hosted parties featuring skits and plays, and who generally lightened the serious tone of academic medicine practiced at a demanding level, Seldin engendered a warm spirit of camaraderie in his department. The piles of reprints, books, articles and photos that clutter his office floor are replete with warm tributes from his students, residents and faculty colleagues.

Seldin's desire to assemble a prestigious full-time faculty posed a formidable challenge. Not only were departmental funds for recruiting limited, but he had precious little in the way of space and equipment for research. "We started out [in 1952] with an annual budget of about $20,000," he related. "Perhaps it was increased a few thousand by eliminating the lecture stipends."[1] Having wisely come to the considered conclusion that it would be difficult to attract a high caliber group of established physician scientists to a school with such limited resources, he began to look within. "I simply couldn't afford to recruit from the outside. So I began to groom research fellows and junior faculty from the best students at Southwestern. A research program was instituted in which third year students worked in my laboratory in the shacks. The

SCUTPUPPY PRODUCTIONS
PRESENTS THE 1987 SENIOR CLASS IN

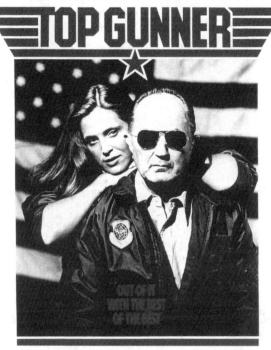

Don Seldin in a playful mood, here "starring" as the "top gunner" in a senior medical student film.

best and brightest were sent to the National Institutes of Health for training in clinical research after they graduated from medical school, and were then brought back to Dallas and appointed to the faculty."[3]

Over the years, this strategy paid huge dividends. In just seven years the faculty in the Department of Internal Medicine grew from three to forty full-time individuals. In a remarkably short time the department took its place among the best in the country—and it never looked back. "All these individuals did research and teaching, yet none of them were brought here to only carry out research. Similarly, nobody was brought here solely to do clinical work. They were all in the flexible model of the clinical scholar in various sub-specialty areas. I wanted everybody to be comfortable in practicing and teaching general internal medicine no matter what his or her specialty was. But in addition, all of them were expected to be involved in some specialty area of clinical medicine, and all were required to do research."[1]

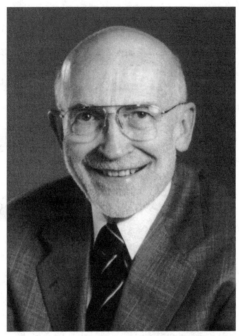

Jean Wilson, long-time faculty member in the Department of Internal Medicine at UT Southwestern. Dr. Wilson was elected to the U.S. National Academy of Sciences in 1983.

Jean Wilson is a prominent example of one of Seldin's early homegrown successes. Born and raised in Texas, Wilson hailed from a Methodist background and aspired to becoming a medical missionary. Before attending medical school, his imagination was fired by reading *Arrowsmith*, Sinclair Lewis's famous novel about a doctor who entered medical research in order to contribute to humankind. Wilson was admitted to UT Southwestern early after Seldin's arrival. "The University of Texas at Austin [where Wilson attended college] had a beautiful campus," he related. "So it was an incredible shock to see the shacks and to attend classes in an old filling station."[8] Nor was he particularly stimulated by the heavy dose of didactic teaching that comprised the first two years at medical school, a period focused mainly on the basic sciences, with no exposure to clinical medicine.

> I am not certain why I decided to stick it out. But within a few weeks of starting the third [clinical] year it was clear that I had made the right decision. The clinical experience was thrilling.... [Much of] the reason for this dramatic change was my encounter with Seldin. He

was a dynamic and enthusiastic educator and a brilliant clinician, and he instilled in me the belief that academic medicine is the highest of callings…. My decision was strengthened when I spent the summer of 1954 as a student research fellow in [his] laboratory studying the effects of adrenal hormones on acid-base balance in rats.[9]

Seldin quickly cast Wilson's career path in the physician-scientist training mold. After graduating from medical school, Wilson remained in Dallas as an intern and resident in internal medicine, continuing his clinical research under Seldin and later under Marvin Siperstein, another of Seldin's stellar faculty recruits. A renowned investigator in diabetes and cholesterol metabolism, Siperstein trained and inspired several generations of physician-scientists, and over the years he mentored a number of young UT Southwestern faculty and research fellows, including the illustrious duo of Brown and Goldstein. In 1958 Wilson gained a precious commission in the U.S. Public Health Service and moved to the NIH for two years of research training. Immediately thereafter he joined the faculty in the Department of Internal Medicine, where he has remained. In 1983 Jean Wilson was elected to membership at the U.S. Na-

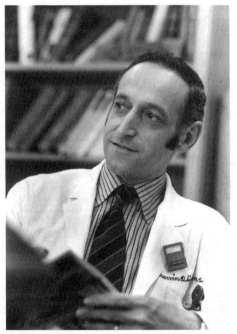

Marvin Siperstein, an expert in cholesterol metabolism and an important early mentor to Mike Brown and Joe Goldstein.

tional Academy of Sciences, the fourth UT Southwestern faculty member to be so honored.

Seldin employed all manner of creative strategies to promote his fledgling program in internal medicine. Capitalizing on his professional (and often personal) relationships with leaders in academic medicine around the country, he instituted an exchange program between chief residents in internal medicine at the Harvard teaching hospitals and Southwestern. A classic example of his entrepreneurship is revealed when he was once approached by a group of Dallas citizens interested in helping patients with rheumatoid arthritis. "Their idea was to build some sort of mobile unit with a nurse who would go around and offer physiotherapy and other forms of medical care to patients with rheumatic disease. But I was able to persuade them that their money would be much more wisely spent on adding a new clinical research program in rheumatology."[3] This initiative facilitated Seldin's recruitment of the celebrated rheumatologist Morris Ziff to the department.

✵ ✵ ✵ ✵ ✵

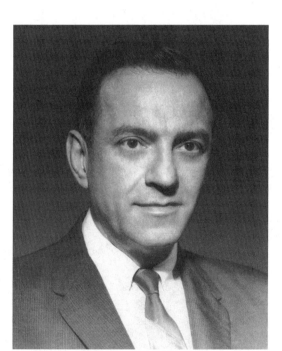

Morris Ziff, a renowned rheumatologist, joined the Department of Internal Medicine at Southwestern Medical School in 1958.

Burton Combes, another long time member of the faculty of the Department of Internal Medicine, joined Seldin's rapidly expanding faculty in 1957. Like Seldin, he came to Dallas site unseen. Intent on securing an academic position, Combes wrote to a number of U.S. institutions while in England for a year of postgraduate training. "The one person who responded immediately was Don Seldin. Other places, including San Francisco and Denver, were very constipated in their responses and that put me off. My wife and I knew that Dallas was growing and that it was a place considered to have promise. And we knew that there was a medical school there. But we knew very little about Southwestern itself. It was Seldin's attentiveness and responsiveness that brought me to Dallas. When I arrived I found an absolutely spectacular group here."[10]

> When I saw the shacks I thought, 'Oh my God, what have I got myself into?' The floors were undulating and when it rained the undulations would fill up with water. But these puddles were easily remedied. One simply drilled a hole in the floor and the water drained out! Seriously, though, the bottom line was Seldin. He was magnetic. He absolutely insisted on excellence and he surrounded himself with excellent and stimulating people. We all did research, but we were all required to be physicians and to attend on the wards.
>
> I especially recall the intense meetings we would have when any of us were preparing to present our work at national meetings, particularly the meetings of the American Society for Clinical Investigation. There was a lot of pride associated with being invited to present talks at national or even regional meetings and a huge effort was expended in making these talks first rate. Seldin insisted on this and put his heart and soul into every one of them.
>
> The question is often asked, 'How did this unknown entity in Dallas succeed so well?' Well, in my view we didn't have a past to define how we should operate. We also had a lot of very bright people who wanted to be successful and it was a time in academic medicine when if you were motivated you could get financial support to do your own research. And Don fostered all of this to the maximum. He set extremely high standards, but if you could meet these standards you took huge pride in what was happening.[10]

Other members of the department echoed these sentiments. Daniel (Dan) Foster, who succeeded Seldin as the chairman of Internal Medicine and was a classmate of Wilson; John Fordtran, a distinguished gastroenterologist; Michael Brown; and Joseph Goldstein all voiced the same plaudits. They painted a picture of a magnetic, intense individual with an astonishing com-

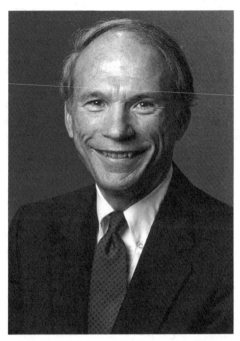

Daniel Foster succeeded Don Seldin as Chairman of the Department of Internal medicine and served in that capacity from 1988–2003.

mand of clinical medicine—a man with exacting standards who could stir terror in the souls of students, interns, and residents, but a man with compassion and devotion and an unwavering commitment to clinical teaching and research. Mike Brown recalled an example of Seldin's resolve.

> In the late '60s and early '70s there was a huge anti-intellectual movement among students at the University of Pennsylvania [where Brown attended medical school] and elsewhere of course. So much so, that a day in the spring that used to be set aside for research presentations by students at Penn was converted to a 'social· services' day. The students had speakers come through to talk about poverty and other social issues that were in the limelight in the sixties and seventies. When I came to Southwestern I was surprised to find that we were the only major medical center that I knew of without a satellite medical presence in the ghetto areas of the city. Seldin absolutely refused to do this. His position was that he was already running a large service taking care of poor people in a charity county hospital. He said, 'If patients come to Parkland we will give them the very best care that sci-

ence can bring to them. But I will not dilute my faculty by sending them out to work in clinics.' He was not indifferent in the least. On the contrary, he was very concerned about the welfare of the poor. But Seldin wasn't willing to compromise his professional resolve. His position was, 'I strongly encourage the city to establish clinics for the poor. But they need to find other doctors to man them.'[11]

CHAPTER 6

CHARLES CAMERON SPRAGUE—
A MILK-DRINKING TEXAS BOY

Thirty-nine-year-old George Aagaard, the dean appointed in 1951, came from the University of Minnesota with "a reputation as a calm, diplomatic statesman who brought order out of chaos."[1] As John Chapman explains, "[f.]or once Southwestern had a dean who ... had previous administrative experience."[2] Though in Dallas for just three years before being lured away by the University of Washington, another fledgling state medical school seeking national visibility, Aagaard made substantial progress at Southwestern.

The Texas legislature appropriated $2.75 million for the medical school's first permanent building in 1951. When the lowest construction bid came in $100,000 over that figure, however, Aagaard faced a serious dilemma. Unless he could come up with the difference, it would be six months before the matter could be discussed again. Chapman provides a vivid account of Aagaard's solution for this problem.

> At about 10:00 p.m. he fired up his Foundation-provided V-8 and struck [from Austin] for Dallas. The speedometer needle stood rather constantly at 80, except as the numerous towns along the old highway necessitated a somewhat more sedate speed, and by 3:00 a.m. he was back in Dallas for three hours of sleep. Much earlier, one is sure, than had happened in many years, Cary's phone rang. Aagaard was asking at six o'clock in the morning if the [Southwestern Medical] Foundation could provide the additional funds. Cary was no man to permit a young Minnesotan to outdo him. By seven o'clock establishment phones all over Dallas had pulled men out of bed to vote 'yes.' And before noon Aagaard was back in Austin, within the deadline of acceptance [of the bid].[2]

In 1954, Aagaard, with the backing of Governor Shivers, obtained state funds to erect a second building for the clinical sciences. The Edward H. Cary Building for Basic Sciences opened in 1955, and the Hoblitzelle Building for Clinical Sciences, named for Karl Hoblitzelle (Cary's successor as president of the

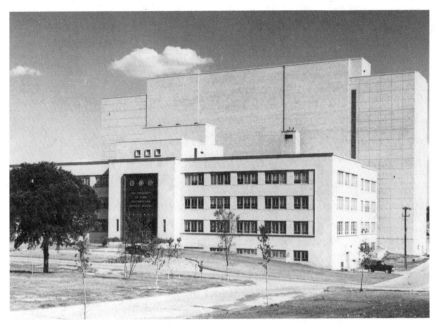

The Edward H. Cary Building for Basic Science (front) and the Hoblitzelle Building for Clinical Sciences (behind) were the first two buildings erected on the new campus site.

Southwestern Medical Foundation and the donor of the property on Harry Hines Boulevard where the new school was located), opened in 1958. The prefabricated shacks were finally abandoned.

John Chapman noted: "By the end of 1955 ... if one looked at Southwestern as it had staggered along six years earlier, it had thrived mightily."[2] However, much remained to be accomplished. Indeed, when in 1956 the president of the University of Texas established the Committee of Seventy-Five to review the strengths and weaknesses of the entire university system, the report on the medical school in Dallas was by no means glowing. "In spite of some solid accomplishments, Southwestern Medical School was not [yet] a distinguished institution."[2]

Seldin agreed. "The Department of Internal Medicine was thriving, but with the possible exception of the Department of Obstetrics and Gynecology, which enjoyed a national reputation under Jack Pritchard's leadership, the other clinical departments were languishing academically and the basic sciences were singularly without distinction. I would have to say that in the early

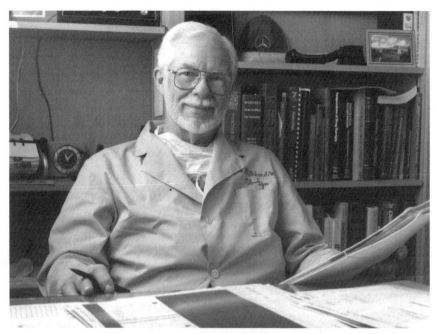

Jack Pritchard chaired the Department of Obstetrics and Gynecology from 1955 to 1969.

1960s the school as a whole was not a strong institution, either at the basic science or clinical levels."[3]

✳ ✳ ✳ ✳ ✳

Seldin, now a prominent national figure in academic medicine, was presented with several opportunities to leave Dallas for "greener pastures"—none of which he ever considered. In 1962, however, he was offered an endowed chair at Harvard University with directorship of the Department of Internal Medicine at the Beth Israel Hospital. This was an attractive offer by any standards, and for a while Seldin was uncertain whether or not he would stay in Dallas. "I tried to keep this as quiet as possible, but everybody became aware of the situation and I had a number of people come by to indicate how anxious they were that I would stay."[3] Much to his surprise (and subsequent delight), one of his visitors was the chancellor of the University of Texas at Austin, Harry Huntt Ransom.

Ransom had succeeded Logan Wilson as chancellor of the University of Texas, having previously served as president. Perhaps best remembered for amassing a vast library collection, which is now housed in the Harry Ransom

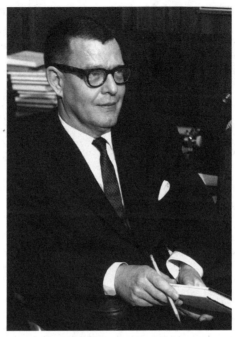

Harry Huntt Ransom (1908–1976), chancellor of the University of Texas and the most significant library builder in the university's history. The Harry Ransom Center houses one of the most distinguished libraries in the world.

Humanities Center at UT Austin and is considered one of the world's great libraries, Harry Ransom was dedicated to unqualified academic excellence. As noted by John Chapman:

> Under Ransom's direction the university as a whole began to move into its present day form. While for many years [it] had occupied a respectable position among state universities, it was not one of the truly distinguished schools of the United States. As a result of [Logan] Wilson's initial efforts, but especially during Ransom's persuasive guidance, the university undertook to realize its program of excellence. All branches and all departments began to aspire to greatness and within a period of about ten years the University of Texas surged forward in relation to many other state universities. For once the government of the state, the board of regents, and the administration of the university seemed united in an effort to produce a great university. Everybody began to talk about a 'critical mass' of faculty.[2]

Seldin described his meeting with Ransom.

> To this day I don't know who orchestrated that visit. Ransom came
> up to Dallas and talked to me about remaining here. We had a long
> discussion during which I highlighted the major weaknesses and
> strengths of the school as I saw them. I told him that I thought the
> Department of Internal Medicine was doing well, but I didn't think
> the medical school in Dallas would advance as a major academic in-
> stitution if the clinical sciences in just one department achieved aca-
> demic dignity. I also mentioned the weaknesses in the basic sciences.
> Ransom listened attentively. He essentially told me that he wouldn't
> put financial resources into the school by way of a blank check. But
> if the school took the initiative to request well thought out programs,
> appointments and activities, he would support them to the full.[3]

Seldin was impressed that the highest administrative official in the University of Texas System had taken the trouble to visit and communicate with him
directly. Once again, in the final analysis he felt optimistic about what the future might hold for the medical school in Dallas—and he decided to stay.

Improvements came slowly but steadily. By the time that Aagaard's successor, former chairman of the Department of Pathology, Atticus James (Jim) Gill
ended his tenure as dean in 1967, a third medical school building named for
another prominent benefactor, Dan Danciger, was completed. This building
not only added new office and research laboratory space, it also physically linked
the medical school to Parkland Hospital, promoting easy back and forth between the hospital's clinical wards and the medical school's research laboratories. The school's annual budget had also grown—from a mere $500,000 in
1949 to a substantial $10 million in 1967, and "it could be said of Southwest-
ern in 1965–66 that it was generally recognized as being a very good medical
school."[2] Still, it was by no means in the major leagues, and could not yet legitimately consider itself a peer of institutions such as the medical schools at
Harvard, Yale, Stanford, or the other top tier schools.

* * * * *

Jim Gill was well respected by the Texas legislature and the Dallas community. As a result, he succeeded in bringing needed financial and managerial
stability to the medical school. However, he was considered by many in the
faculty to be philosophically conservative with respect to the expected rate of
growth and development. In 1965, several faculty leaders had become sufficiently restless about the pace of the school's progress that they held a retreat
in Salado, Texas, at which they overwhelmingly agreed that aggressive aca-

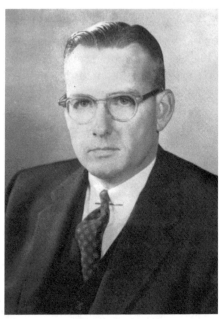

Atticus James (A.J.) Gill served as Chairman of the Department of Pathology from 1943 to 1967 and as Dean of the Medical School from 1955–1967.

demic growth should be a priority for Southwestern Medical School. In 1967, after serving thirteen years as dean, Gill resigned.

After much deliberation a committee to identify Gill's successor recommended the dean of Tulane University Medical School, Charles (Charlie) Cameron Sprague. Sprague hailed from a prominent Dallas family. Indeed, his father George Sprague served as mayor of the city from 1937–39. Charlie Sprague completed his undergraduate studies at Southern Methodist University (SMU), where he excelled both in the classroom and on the playing field. He was an All Southwest Conference tackle in football, and captain of SMU's 1936 Rose Bowl team. He also captained the SMU basketball team and participated in track and field.

Midway through his junior year a football injury prompted Sprague to seek medical assistance—purportedly the first time he had ever entered a doctor's office. According to Sprague, this encounter piqued his interest in medicine. He obtained his medical training at the University of Texas Medical Branch in Galveston, declining the opportunity to attend the Baylor College of Medicine in Dallas because it was considerably more expensive. Following an internship at the U.S. Naval Medical Center in Bethesda and residency training at Tulane University School of Medicine, Sprague was named a fellow and instructor at

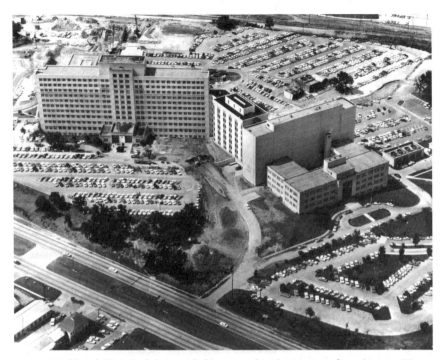

A new Parkland Hospital (upper left) opened at its present location on Harry Hines Boulevard in 1954 and continued to serve as the exclusive teaching hospital for the medical school. The Cary and Hoblitzelle buildings are shown in the right foreground. The Dan Danciger Building links them to the hospital.

Tulane, where he established a division of hematology. Not too much later Sprague was awarded fellowships to study hematology, first at Washington University in St. Louis, and then at Oxford University School of Medicine in England. He returned to Tulane in 1952 as assistant professor and director of the hematology laboratory. He was named full professor in 1962, and was appointed Dean of the Medical School the following year.

A member of the search committee for a new dean at Southwestern Medical School, Seldin enthusiastically courted Sprague. An article written shortly after Sprague's death in 2005 revealed that Dallas business leaders were equally enthusiastic. "Some of the most powerful men in Dallas—James Aston, head of Republic Bank and treasurer of the Southwest Medical Foundation; Mayor J. Erik Jonsson and his co-founders of Texas Instruments, Cecil Green and Eugene McDermott; developer John Stemmons; and George MacGregor, then president of the medical foundation—had lunch with Dr. Sprague at the Petroleum Club."[4] James Aston "later recalled [that while Sprague] was trying to

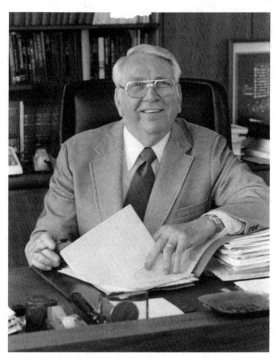

Charles Cameron Sprague (1916–2005) served as Dean of the Medical School from 1967–1972 and as the first President of the University of Texas Southwestern Medical Center at Dallas from 1972–1986.

persuade us that he was the man for the job, we were trying to persuade him to leave the job at Tulane."[4]

"Charlie was an outstanding dean,"[3] Seldin commented. "Everybody loved him—with good reason. He possessed huge warmth and congeniality and was an effective spokesman for the school. He was never devious; he was never contrived. Charlie was the proverbial milk-drinking Texas boy. Even though his background and experience was in clinical medicine, he was very much in favor of developing the basic sciences and promoted them vigorously."[3]

Sprague was an experienced administrator with national visibility. "Already high in the councils of the Association of American Medical Colleges, he was clearly slated to become president [of the association]."[2] For nineteen years, Sprague served Southwestern Medical School as dean and then as its first president. Under his leadership, the institution truly came of age. "When I arrived here in 1967, this institution was an adolescent, although an adolescent whose character already was apparent,"[5] he said near the end of his career. "But what was then a somewhat malnourished child, poorly clothed, is now a vigorous, robust and healthy adult."[5]

Recognizing full well that attracting distinguished leaders required distinguished physical facilities, Sprague had overseen a major building program at Tulane. New buildings, therefore, were high on his priority list at Southwestern. He was also aware of the need to strengthen the basic sciences. "There was a clear understanding on the part of virtually everyone that the major initial thrust ought to be to strengthen the basic sciences, both in terms of providing additional much-needed space and also to recruit outstanding people into these departments."[5] "With immense energy Sprague turned his first attention to the problems of construction and within a year offered a general plan of development to be undertaken in two phases. The first phase included the construction and completion of buildings that were essential to the development of prominent departments in the basic sciences, extension of space for research laboratories of the clinical sciences, the construction of a library building, and the provision of adequate lecture and seminar rooms for the increased classes of the future."[2] This massive program, the concept of which had been presented to the board of regents of the University of Texas under Gill's tenure as dean, would more than double the campus size (with close to a million square feet of new space). Seldin's desire to strengthen the basic sciences complemented Sprague's enthusiasm. The two men forged a formidable partnership based on mutual respect and a shared vision.

Sprague's building plan carried a price tag of about $40 million. Fortunately, the federal government was still supporting building projects through the NIH granting system and a $21 million building proposal was successfully steered through the NIH (the last of the NIH largesse in that arena). The State of Texas, too, provided funds. At the end of the day, however, Sprague still needed $7.5 million. Once again, the Southwestern Medical Foundation stepped in, launching a fundraising effort in the Dallas community that exceeded this goal by almost a million dollars.

The only constraint that Sprague placed on the architects "was that all the buildings be physically connected to each other and to Parkland hospital, to promote easy access between different groups and departments."[5] This philosophy of erecting academic buildings with horizontal contiguity on every floor was strictly adhered to over the years. It is no accident that one can now walk about half a mile from the Children's Medical Center to the McDermott Plaza on the main campus without having to step outside (some walk the route for exercise in the hot summer months). In subsequent years, this design was reiterated on the new North Campus, joining six buildings into a single monolith of about two million square feet.

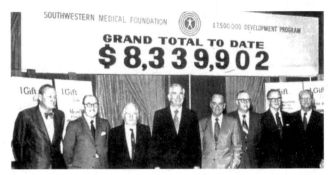

The Southwest Medical Foundation contributed over $8M in a fund raising campaign to help capital improvements at the medical school. Leaders in the campaign included (from left to right) John M. Stemmons, George L. MacGregor, Eugene McDermott, Dr. Charles Sprague, Joe M. Dealey, Lloyd Bowles, Dr. C. F. Hamilton and Dan C. Williams.

With the completion of space for the basic sciences, Sprague set about recruiting academic leaders to upgrade the Departments of Physiology, Biochemistry, Microbiology & Immunology, and Cell Biology. All were people of exceptional academic distinction who, like Seldin, recognized the school's potential, and all were eager to have the opportunity to place their individual stamps on its programs.

※ ※ ※ ※ ※

Coincidentally, the first two appointments involved two prominent scientists from the same institution—the University of Pennsylvania. In 1965, Samuel (Don) McCann was appointed chairman of the Department of Physiology. Soon after, Ronald (Ron) Estabrook joined Southwestern Medical School as chairman of the Department of Biochemistry. "When these two individuals were recruited here, they instantly became among the most famous scientists on this campus,"[6] Jean Wilson explained. Their academic reputations were such that in 1979 Estabrook became the first UT Southwestern faculty member to be elected to the U.S. National Academy of Sciences.

McCann had built his scientific reputation as an outstanding neuroendocrinologist. An article published in the late 1990s entitled *Forty Years of Neuroendocrinology: A Tribute to S. M. McCann* made reference to "the strength and vigor of McCann's research, which over forty-five years evolved into a coherent body of knowledge that integrates various key concepts of biology into testable hypotheses, generating work that is conceptually novel and of profound physiological and medical relevance."[7] McCann is credited with "ex-

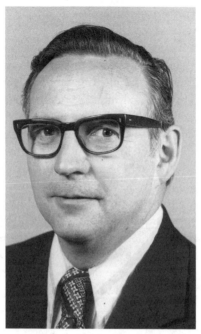

Ron Estabrook chaired the Department of Biochemistry and also served as the first Dean of the Graduate School. In 1979 Estabrook became the first UT Southwestern faculty member to be elected to the U.S. National Academy of Sciences.

panding the frontiers of existing knowledge in neuroendocrinology with a body of work that included over 650 original manuscripts."[7] "It was said by some that his department did not have sufficient breadth,"[6] Wilson commented. "But there is no question that Don McCann attracted a number of outstanding people to work on neuroendocrinology in his department."[6] The 1977 Nobel Prize in Medicine or Physiology was awarded to Roger Guillemin, Andrew Schally, and Rosalyn Yalow for their discoveries concerning peptide hormone production in the brain. Many believed that McCann had been unfairly passed over—and that he never forgot this perceived slight. McCann remained chairman of the Department of Physiology until 1985, when he was succeeded by James Stull.

※ ※ ※ ※ ※

Ron Estabrook, a biophysicist by training, had risen rapidly through the academic ranks at the University of Pennsylvania and was on the short list at a number of schools seeking new leadership in the field. Estabrook worked closely with the renowned biophysicist Britton Chance, director of the Johnson Foundation for Medical Physics at the University of Pennsylvania. Though keen on building his own academic program, none of the many offers he received excited him—until he visited UT Southwestern. "I recall that the school was having a difficult time recruiting a new chairman for biochemistry in the mid and late 1960s.... This was not too long after the Kennedy assassination and many people didn't want to come to Dallas for that reason. Dallas was blacklisted."[8]

There is little question that the Kennedy assassination negatively impacted the perception of Dallas by outsiders, and that this perception in turn impacted recruiting efforts. Jean Wilson pointed out that around the time of the 1960 presidential elections, several hate groups plagued Dallas politics. "Furthermore, its reputation for extremism was fostered by a rabid editorial policy in both daily newspapers. Paradoxically, however, the assassination had a long-term beneficial effect on the city because this tragic event eventually mobilized more rational and tolerant attitudes in the city."[6] In the same vein, Steve McKnight, the present chairman of biochemistry, related a revealing anecdote of those difficult times for the city of Dallas.

> A former faculty member once told me that somewhere around 1965 he went to a meeting in Chicago. He took a cab from the airport and the cab driver asked where he was from. The faculty member replied 'I'm from Dallas.' The cab driver pulled over on the freeway and abruptly said, 'Get out!' Why did Los Angeles not get blamed for Bobby Kennedy getting killed there? In fact, I don't think Memphis got blamed for the assassination of Martin Luther King. But Dallas was somehow blamed for Jack Kennedy being killed here. I think it's only in the last decade or so that the city no longer bears that burden.[9]

Fortunately, Estabrook was not influenced by these recent political events.

> I received a call from Marvin Siperstein on behalf of the search committee, who suggested that I at least come down and take a look at UT Southwestern. As soon as I met Charlie Sprague I became a great admirer. He is the primary reason I came to Southwestern. He was the sort of man one fell in love with as soon as one met him. He described his vision of developing the basic sciences and this excited me enormously. He immediately invited me to come up with a five-year plan for the Department of Biochemistry. Some people find this hard to believe, but when I accepted the position I trusted Charlie so completely I never asked for or received a formal letter detailing the terms

of my appointment. Eventually, he gave me everything I asked for. [It is worth pointing out that over the years the "hard to believe" notion of accepting the responsibility of rebuilding an academic department at UT Southwestern on a handshake agreement of promised resources has satisfied many others, regardless of who was dean at the time.] I was also deeply impressed by the commitment that I observed from the Dallas community. Charlie had a dinner for me on my first visit and introduced me to people from the Southwestern Medical Foundation. It was clear that they were very supportive of the initiative to build strong basic sciences at Southwestern. I'd been looking at chairmanships in a number of places around the country, including at the University of Pennsylvania. But none of them impressed me as much as the combination of Charlie Sprague's vision and the physical and financial resources that Southwestern offered.[8]

During his fourteen-year tenure as chairman of the Biochemistry Department, Estabrook built a world-recognized center for biochemical research (in particular that related to the cytochrome P450 system, a biochemical system that is fundamental in detoxifying drugs and other foreign compounds introduced into our bodies). He was elected to the U.S. National Academy of Sciences in 1979, the first UT Southwestern faculty member to be so honored. In 1981, he received an honorary doctor of medicine degree from the Karolinska Institute in Sweden, and in 1999 he received the George Scott Award from the Toxicology Forum, an international non-profit organization devoted to promoting open dialogue among the various segments of society concerned with toxicology. In the spring of 2006, a symposium at UT Southwestern entitled "Celebration of Biochemistry" recognized the contributions of Estabrook and his long-time faculty colleague John M. Johnston to both the medical school and the field of biochemistry.

* * * * *

Soon after Estabrook's arrival in Dallas, it was decided that the Department of Anatomy would be converted to the Department of Cellular Biology. Several prominent cell biologists were considered to lead this endeavor, among them Estabrook's colleague at the University of Pennsylvania, Rupert E. Billingham. A pioneer in the fields of reproductive immunology and organ transplantation, Billingham was chairman of the Department of Medical Genetics in the School of Medicine at Penn. As a graduate student, he had studied at Oxford University with Nobel laureate Sir Peter Medawar, and had moved with Medawar to the University of Birmingham to carry out seminal

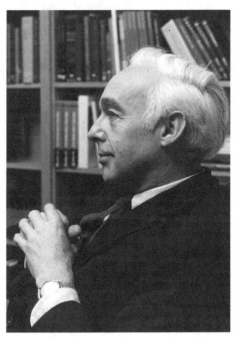

Rupert E. Billingham (1921–2002) was a distinguished immunologist and cell biologist who chaired the Department of Cell Biology from 1971–1986. Billingham was a fellow of the Royal Society of London.

studies in transplantation biology. When Medawar was awarded the 1960 Nobel Prize in Physiology or Medicine for the discovery of acquired immunological tolerance (together with MacFarlin Burnett), he graciously shared the prize money with his former student. Many thought that Billingham should have also shared in the formal award.

Seldin recalled how his experience in recruiting Billingham to UT Southwestern was easier than he feared.

> I remember that one night Marvin Siperstein and I were in a restaurant talking about recruiting Billingham. I initially considered that absolutely ridiculous. Billingham was an immunologist of the highest order. Why would he want to come to Dallas to take over the Department of Anatomy, where there was no cell biology at all? But Marvin thought it was worth a try. What could we lose? Subsequently I learned that Billingham and the chairman of the Department of Medicine at the University of Pennsylvania were at odds and I became more intrigued. Ultimately the search committee approached Billing-

ham and I think he accepted the job within a week or two. I was flabbergasted, because I regarded Billingham as a giant in basic science. No one understood why he didn't share the Nobel Prize with Medawar. It was an absolutely sensational recruitment.[3]

Billingham brought with him from Philadelphia the distinguished immunologist Wayne Streilein and contributed cutting edge immunological research as chairman of the Department of Cell Biology from 1971 until his retirement in 1986. Like his later English counterpart in biochemistry, Joe Sambrook, Billingham was an elected Fellow of the Royal Society, the formal equivalent of the U.S. National Academy of Sciences.

* * * * *

Jonathan Uhr, who succeeded Edward Sulkin as chairman of the Department of Microbiology, was Seldin's fourth key basic science recruit. Uhr was director of the Irvington House Institute for Rheumatic Fever and Allied Diseases (affiliated with the New York University Medical Center) when it fell on hard times

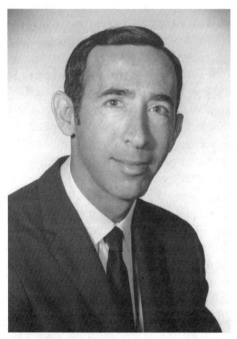

Jonathan Uhr chaired the Department of Microbiology from 1972–1998 and developed one of the premier centers of immunology in the country. Uhr was elected to the U.S. National Academy of Sciences in 1993.

in the early 1970s. When Seldin heard of this critical "push factor," he contacted Uhr directly. Like Estabrook and Billingham, Uhr had never visited Southwestern, but was aware of the reputation of its Department of Internal Medicine. "I was on the committee at New York University that interviewed perspective interns for the Department of Medicine. We were well aware then that graduates from Southwestern were front rank in terms of clinical medicine. They were equivalent to graduates from anywhere in the country."[10] Uhr was impressed and excited by his first visit to Southwestern Medical School.

> A new building was being erected and it was clear that I would be able to move into it within a year if I came here. I was also offered the opportunity to fill about a dozen new faculty positions. The existing department was virtually empty, so I saw a fabulous opportunity to build something of distinction. Frankly I was ready to be an academic chairman and I wanted to build a front rank department. Southwestern was a very attractive place at which to realize these ambitions. In addition, I frankly liked the idea of coming to Texas. I was impressed by the friendliness and the openness of the people, the likes of which I had not encountered in New York. I had examined job offers in Chicago, Pittsburgh, San Diego and Berkeley. They simply weren't comparable as far as I was concerned.[10]

> That time in the early 1970s was a major turning point for the school. It was not really well known then. It had superb clinical departments and a few solid basic science departments, but not ones with national reputations. Under the guidance of Charlie Sprague the clinical departments had agreed to mount a huge effort to obtain front rank basic science departments; a very institutionally motivated gesture and a very unselfish one. The Department of Medicine was so cramped for space that they had equipment spilling all over the hallways. Yet here they were supporting building beautiful new laboratories for the basic sciences. Don Seldin not only created an extraordinary Department of Internal Medicine, but was also very strong in the belief that basic science and clinical medicine absolutely must to be wedded. This was not the attitude at many other places. This was the Vietnam era and the time of the counter-culture revolution and the value of basic science was being questioned by young people all over the country. But Seldin held fast to his views and I give him a great deal of credit for this turning point in the school's history.[10]

An avid tennis player, Uhr was also not at all displeased with the sunny Dallas climate. He built an outstanding Department of Microbiology that became widely recognized as one of the finest in the country. At one time, his faculty included several luminaries in immunology, including Jan Klein (presently at Pennsylvania State University) and Donald Capra (now at the University of Oklahoma). Ellen Vitetta, another distinguished faculty member in Uhr's department, was the first woman from UT Southwestern to be elected to the U.S. National Academy of Sciences (in 1994). She now directs the Cancer Immunology Center. Uhr was elected to the National Academy in 1984, and to the American Academy of Arts and Sciences in 1993.

✳ ✳ ✳ ✳ ✳

By the mid-1970s, the UT Southwestern Medical School had garnered a solid national reputation and was probably ranked in the top third of American medical schools (this was long before the days when a popular news magazine took it upon itself to determine the rankings of academic institutions.) To effectively capitalize on its growing visibility, the last thing the school needed was another name change! However, the Board of Regents of the University of Texas System wanted uniformity among its various medical centers, and in 1972 the school's name was changed to the University of Texas Health Science Center at Dallas. The word "center" underscored the institution's changing scope—aside from a medical school, there was now a graduate school and a School of Allied Health Sciences. Around the same time, an Office of the President was created (in addition to those of the deans of each school). Sprague was appointed the first president, and a year later Fred Bonte became the new dean of the medical school, a position he occupied until 1980, when he was succeeded by Kern Wildenthal, dean of the graduate school.

With the rebuilding of the Departments of Biochemistry, Cell Biology, and Microbiology well in hand, attention was shifted to another fundamental bastion of basic science in any first rate medical school, the Department of Pharmacology. The search committee quickly focused on Alfred (Al) G. Gilman at the University of Virginia, a leading figure in modern pharmacology. Joe Goldstein, a member of the search committee, contacted Gilman sometime in the late 1970s. He and Gilman had been postdoctoral fellows in the same laboratory at the NIH a decade earlier, and Goldstein held him in high esteem. But Gilman had no interest in the position. Not only was he deeply involved with his research program, which would later yield him a Nobel Prize, he was also writing the 6th edition of his father's famous pharmacology textbook *The Pharmacological Basis of Therapeutics*. "I was working my tail off on the book and was much too busy to even think about a new job," Gilman related.[11]

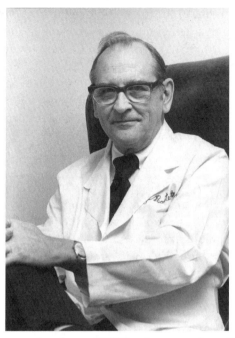

Fred Bonte served as dean of UT Southwestern from 1973–1980.

The search committee approached several other nationally prominent scientists, including Martin Rodbell, a distinguished investigator at the NIH who was later to be Gilman's co-recipient of the 1994 Nobel prize. Rodbell initially accepted the position, and then changed his mind at the last minute for personal reasons. Gilman is of course fully aware of (and more than slightly amused by) the fact that both future recipients of the Nobel Prize in Physiology or Medicine were recruited to the same position at UT Southwestern! He related an anecdote that transpired a few years after he declined Goldstein's initial overture. "Sometime in the autumn of 1980 I was at a meeting with Marty [Rodbell] and he was regaling everyone with incredible stories about how lavishly Dallas had recruited him. He was recounting what a fantastic place it was, and so on, and I remember thinking that maybe I shouldn't have terminated that initial phone call so quickly!"[11] Indeed, when UT Southwestern contacted Gilman a second time following Rodbell's withdrawal, his recollections of what Rodbell had said about the institution made him more attentive. "When Joe Goldstein first called me I knew just about nothing about Southwestern. But Rodbell's account sort of set the stage because he described the place so glowingly."[1] Wildenthal, now dean of the medical school, assigned Seldin the task of once again approaching

Gilman, an encounter that the then rising star at the University of Virginia readily recalls.

> I had never met Don, but I had certainly heard of him. When my assistant told me that Dr. Seldin from Southwestern Medical School was on the phone I knew immediately what the call was going to be about. Don introduced himself very graciously, saying, 'Dr. Gilman, would you please give me just fifteen minutes of your time to describe the situation here.' I didn't know then what fifteen minutes meant to Don Seldin. But I don't think I got to say another word for about an hour! He laid it all out on the phone. He had all his ducks lined up. Every square inch of space, every nickel of funds was mentioned. He did a magnificent job of recruiting me—just on the phone. I told him that I would talk to my wife Kathy. She was then a tutor of dyslexic children and as it turned out there were good opportunities for her in Dallas. After that things happened very quickly. I abhor long drawn out job-seeking affairs. So I told the search committee that if we could continue discussions in the same up-front, forthright manner as my discussion with Dr. Seldin I would be happy to take a look at the position. I made a visit in December of 1980 and saw Southwestern for the first time. I made a second visit in January of 1981 with Kathy, and I accepted the job the following month.[11]

✳ ✳ ✳ ✳ ✳

Al Gilman never considered a career other than as a scientist. His father, Alfred Gilman, an eminent academic pharmacologist, is perhaps best known for the famous textbook on pharmacology that he and Louis Goodman initiated while at Yale. (Al Gilman's middle name is Goodman, after his father's collaborator.) Goodman and Gilman ushered in the modern era of cancer chemotherapy with their studies on the effects of nitrogen mustard (mustard gas) on cancer in mice, and later in humans. "The first human patient was someone terminally ill with lymphoma,"[11] Al Gilman related. "She was moribund and they gave her nitrogen mustard and her tumor literally melted. It was an enormous success." These studies, carried out during World War II, were classified because mustard gas was being evaluated for possible use in chemical warfare. Gilman senior and his colleagues, therefore, could not publish their results until the war was over.

> My dad took me fishing a lot—and he took me to his lab a lot. He did a great job of exposing me to science in a fun way. I especially re-

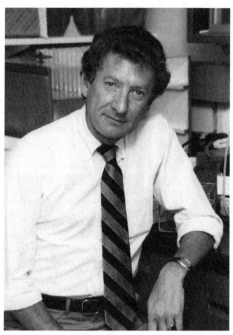

Al Gilman circa 1980. Gilman, Chairman of the Department of Pharmacology from 1981–2005, built one of the premier departments in the country. He was elected to the U.S. National Academy of Sciences in 1986, and won the Nobel Prize in 1994 (see page 4).

member the times when he had to set up special dog heart and lung preparations for the medical students at Columbia University and later at Albert Einstein (where Gilman senior was the founding chairman of the Department of Pharmacology). It took hours of meticulous surgery to prepare these animals and hook them up to these enormous smoked drums [called kymographs], on which a stylus recorded heart and lung activity. I used to watch them doing this surgery and was intrigued with science at an early age.[11]

Gilman went to high school at the Taft School in Watertown, Connecticut,[12] where he "learned how to learn. The education there was superb. The chemistry, physics and math were extraordinary and I was required to write an essay every week."[11] A triumphant back-handed validation of his budding interest in science came on an occasion when his demanding English teacher returned one of his essays with the comment, "'Not bad, Gilman. It still sounds like a lab report, but not bad.'"[11]

Gilman attended Yale University as an undergraduate, and spent much of his senior year in a research laboratory.

> I was presented with an extraordinarily ambitious project that I never really made any headway with. I was asked to consider proving Francis Crick's adaptor hypothesis. [Francis Crick, who, together with Jim Watson, would soon win the Nobel Prize for deciphering the structure of DNA, had hypothesized how the genetic code dictated the correct assembly of specific amino acids into proteins. He correctly postulated the existence in cells of an "adaptor" molecule that was subsequently shown to be an entity called transfer RNA.] Of course I didn't get anywhere with this project, but it was fun thinking about it. It took several major research laboratories several years to solve that one![11]

A series of events led Gilman to medical school at Western Reserve University (now called Case Western Reserve) in Cleveland, Ohio.

> My father had a PhD degree, but he was really a frustrated MD for much of his academic career. His major encouragement to me was that I should get an MD degree and then continue training as a postdoctoral fellow in a basic research lab if I really intended pursuing a research career. Sometime in my junior year at medical school I received a letter from Earl Sutherland, the chairman of pharmacology at Western Reserve. He knew my father well and had told him that he was on the look out for promising young scientists who might be interested in a combined MD, PhD training program that he had recently instituted at Western Reserve. He handpicked every candidate by contacting them personally and he sent me a written invitation to join this seven-year program. I was of course flattered, but seven years sounded like a lifetime to me then—especially to be in Cleveland, Ohio! So I wrote back thanking him but essentially saying, 'No thanks.'
>
> My father didn't push me one way or the other on this issue. But several months later Sutherland wrote to me again saying that he was aware that he had contacted me previously, but wanted to check whether I had had a change of heart. This time he invited me to visit Western Reserve, but indicated that I would have to do so soon as positions in the program were filling up. This time I thought, 'Well what the hell, I'll visit Cleveland and take a look!' So I went out there—and I was enormously impressed. He told me about his interest in understanding how hormones work, and about his discovery of cyclic AMP that he believed was a crucial mediator of hormone action—

but that nobody then was convinced was real. [Sutherland would later win the Nobel Prize for this discovery.] I found this story to be very exciting. Additionally, the new program looked very interesting and I was impressed with the quality of the students who were already re-cruited. I was also not displeased with the amount of the stipend being offered, which I determined I could live on if my girlfriend moved with me and we decided to get married.[11]

Gilman accepted Sutherland's offer, and enrolled in the Western Reserve com-bined MD, PhD degree program. His girlfriend, Kathy Hedland, moved with him to Cleveland, where they were married in due course.

Gilman saw himself as a budding biochemist, not a pharmacologist. More-over, not wanting to precisely emulate his father's career moves, he had reserva-tions about a training program based in a department of pharmacology. When he related his concerns to Sutherland, the man reassuringly patted him on the back and said, "'Al, pharmacology here *is* biochemistry. It's biochemistry with a purpose.' That impressed me a lot. I thought it a wonderful description of mod-ern pharmacology and have used that line myself on many occasions since."[11]

Not long after Gilman enrolled in the graduate program, Sutherland left Western Reserve for a position at Vanderbilt University. By then, Gilman had identified Edward (Ted) Rall, one of Sutherland's collaborators in the cyclic AMP field, as a mentor, and he pursued his Ph.D. thesis research in Rall's laboratory.

In retrospect I was lucky to end up in Rall's laboratory. I had a good friend from Yale whom I told about the program at Western Reserve and he eventually decided to go there as well. When the time came for us to identify a lab to work in we both surveyed all the research laboratories and the two most interesting to both of us were Rall's and the laboratory run by Joe Larner (another Sutherland protégé). Having already worked together at Yale my friend and I decided that we should probably join different research labs. So we decided to flip a coin to determine who would have the first choice. I won the toss and that's how I ended up in Rall's lab.[11]

At this point, it is appropriate to explain the general significance of cyclic AMP in the late 1950s and early 1960s. At the time, little was known about how hormones work. The pervasive dogma among biomedical scientists was that this fundamentally important question was too complicated to address by conventional biochemistry, which involved breaking open cells and tissues to explore what goes on in the extracts. Nor was this attitude restricted to hor-mone research. Enzymology (the study of enzymes, the workhorses in cells) was still something of an infant science, and many biologists had yet to be convinced that the way that enzymes function in intact cells could be accurately mirrored when cells were taken apart. The prevailing notion was that genetics, not biochemistry, would explain how cells really work. As Gilman put it, "Everyone thought that there was something mystical about hormone action that required the use of intact tissues and organs. People believed that the reductionist biochemical approach would never work."[11]

Sutherland and Rall thought otherwise. They were interested in understanding how glycogen is converted to glucose in the liver in response to the hormone adrenaline. It was known that the liver enzyme glycogen phosphorylase, which converts glycogen to glucose, becomes activated in the presence of adrenaline by a factor in liver cell extracts. Sutherland and his colleagues demonstrated that this factor was a compound called cyclic adenosine monophosphate (cyclic AMP), an unusual form of one of the building blocks of adenosine triphosphate (ATP), which is a fundamental source of energy in living cells. It took Sutherland and his group many years to convince the scientific world that the important factor in liver extracts was indeed cyclic AMP, and even longer to prove its then novel cyclic structure. In subsequent years, cyclic AMP was shown to be a mediator of the action of many hormones, and became widely referred to as the "second messenger" (the first messenger being messenger RNA of course, a molecule that conveys "messages" from DNA for the synthesis of proteins in cells). As Gilman stated in his Nobel Prize lecture, "Rall and Sutherland's discovery of cyclic AMP and adenyl cyclase, the hormone-sensitive enzyme that synthesizes the cyclic nucleotide from ATP, gave birth to the concept ... of hormone-regulated synthesis of intracellular second messengers."[13]

Gilman pursued his PhD thesis research on thyroid stimulating hormone. But cyclic AMP was ubiquitous in Rall's laboratory. "I entered the Rall lab, and in over thirty subsequent years I have never escaped the lure of cyclic nucleotide research—despite occasional attempts to try."[13] Gilman fleetingly considered a career in academic clinical medicine, but several desultory experiences with patients confirmed his conviction that he was better suited to the laboratory.

Another attempt to escape the world of cyclic nucleotides came by way of a postdoctoral sojourn with Marshall Nirenberg at the NIH. Gilman was interested in the brain, his curiosity encouraged to some extent by the fact that Rall had been working on cyclic AMP in the brain. He was also struck by the number of prominent molecular biologists who were then moving into neurobiology, widely considered the next frontier of modern biology. For his postdoctoral training, therefore, he looked to the emerging discipline of neurobiology.

The Vietnam War and the attendant threat of the draft motivated many young scientists to explore government service to avoid an unwelcome career interruption. One result of this was that research commissions at the NIH were extremely difficult to come by. But in 1969 Gilman secured a commission in Marshall Nirenberg's laboratory (where he first met Joe Goldstein). Nirenberg had received the Nobel Prize a year earlier for his contributions to deciphering the genetic code and was now trying to understand how nerve cells worked. It is probably more than pure coincidence that Gilman, who would later win a Nobel Prize himself, was mentored by Nobel laureates both as a graduate student and as a post-doctoral research fellow.

Destiny, however, did not allow Gilman to relinquish his involvement with cyclic AMP and second messengers. His discussions with Nirenberg about a research project on nerve cells led to a general consideration of how receptors on the surface of cells recognize and interact with specific signaling molecules (ligands).

> Marshall indicated that the only way that he could think of measuring receptor function was to assay cyclic AMP in these cells under different conditions. He asked me if I knew how to assay cyclic AMP, a brutishly difficult and labor intensive task that sometimes worked and sometimes didn't. It was a horrendous assay to set up. I, and perhaps a half a dozen others in the world were the only ones who knew how to do this. Marshall asked me to describe the assay and immediately recognized how difficult it was going to be. So he suggested an alternative method that I set to thinking about. No sooner did I have a firm grasp on this challenge, with a possible solution in mind, then Marshall came into the lab and said to me, 'I've changed my mind. I don't want you to work on the cyclic AMP assay. I want you to work on learning how to get nerve cells to generate axons when they grow in culture.'[11]

For the next six months, therefore, Gilman worked with nerve cells. "We tried this and we tried that, and eventually we got these nerve cells to grow the way that Marshall wanted them to. But I found this pretty boring and I was constantly thinking about alternative projects. One that eventually surfaced in my mind looked like a potentially really good way of assaying cyclic AMP."[11] So as soon as the nerve cell project was completed and the results published, Gilman set about putting his new assay to the test. "I was convinced that Nirenberg wanted this assay. I certainly knew that the world wanted such an assay. So I went at it enthusiastically. One day, when things were really showing enormous promise, Nirenberg came into the lab and asked me what I was doing. I excitedly told him about my progress with the assay, only to hear that he was still disinterested and wanted me to return to the work on nerve cells."[11] Gilman reluctantly agreed (he had little choice) but made up his mind that he would first complete his work on establishing and perfecting the new assay. Thus began an intense battle of wills. The more Nirenberg nagged Gilman to drop his work on assaying cyclic AMP, the more determined Gilman became to complete the project. "I pleaded with him and pleaded with him. I told him that all I needed was about six weeks and I would have this all done and would then return to the work that he wanted me to pursue."[11] But Nirenberg refused to sanction this interruption and for a while, the two barely spoke.

Gilman did indeed complete his work on the assay almost six weeks later and bravely asked Nirenberg to submit for publication his completed manuscript to the *Proceedings of the National Academy of Sciences,* then (as now) a prestigious scientific journal. [The communication of scientific papers for publication in the *Proceedings* is a privilege granted to members of the National Academy of Sciences. As a member of the Academy, Nirenberg could publish scientific papers of his own, or communicate papers from any other scientist whose work he deemed appropriate for publication in the journal.] Notwithstanding the fact that his laboratory colleagues thought Gilman absolutely crazy to even consider approaching Nirenberg with such a request after the tussle between them, Nirenberg to his credit, recognized the significance of Gilman's work and communicated it to the *Proceedings.* Thus, Gilman's first major contribution to scientific literature was a paper entitled *A Protein Binding Assay for Adenosine 3':5' -Cyclic Monophosphate,* published in November 1970, on which he was the sole author. The latter nuance bears noting, as Nirenberg could have not inappropriately added his own name—most mentors do under such circumstances. As late as the early 1980s, Gilman's paper was one of the ten most frequently cited scientific publications in the world.

In the summer of 1970, Sutherland invited Gilman to present the results of his work at a Gordon Research Conference on cyclic AMP. Gilman was terrified, as any young postdoctoral fellow might be, at the thought of presenting his work to an audience of distinguished senior scientists. But to his pleasure, he received numerous requests for his as yet unpublished manuscript. His career as a scientist was launched; and he began receiving job offers. Ultimately, he accepted a position in the Department of Pharmacology at the University of Virginia under the chairmanship of Joe Larner, yet another Sutherland protégé. Here, Gilman set about deciphering how cyclic AMP worked, an undertaking that ultimately led him into the world of receptors (molecules built into the fabric of cell membranes) that interact with specific extracellular ligands.

Gilman was aware of and closely followed work by Martin Rodbell, who was then at the NIH. Rodbell was the first to reliably isolate preparations of cell membranes loaded with functional receptors. When Rodbell heard Sutherland lecture about cyclic AMP as a "second messenger" in the mid-1960s, he too "turned to the cyclic AMP paradigm [to understand] how hormonal information is transferred across the cell membrane and translated into action [in cells]."[14] This in turn led to his discovery of the importance of a molecule called GTP (functionally related to ATP) in signaling across the cell membrane.

The arrival of Elliot Ross as a postdoctoral fellow in Gilman's laboratory spawned a set of crucial studies designed to understand hormone-sensitive cyclic AMP systems, a challenge that had confounded many biochemists because cell membranes were extremely difficult to work with. Employing a clever combination of genetics and biochemistry, heroic efforts (and good fortune) led to the discovery of a novel membrane-bound protein eventually called G_s that bound GTP. So-called G-proteins had arrived. It was during this hectic and intense period that Gilman was contacted by his former postdoctoral colleague Joe Goldstein, who invited him to consider the chairmanship of the Department of Pharmacology at UT Southwestern.

We now know that G proteins, of which there are multiple forms, are integral components of hormone receptors in cell membranes, and undergo specific changes that are in turn fundamental to numerous aspects of cell signaling, ranging from hormone action to the biochemistry of vision to the generation of the bacterial toxin that causes cholera. The importance of Gilman's and Rodbell's contributions was aptly captured in the presentation speech by a member of the Nobel Committee at the Nobel Prize ceremonies in December 1994.

> The cooperation between the individual building blocks in our body, our cells, runs so smoothly in every possible situation that we seldom have cause to reflect on what a tremendously sophisticated communication system is required. The cells communicate with each other using chemical signals, such as hormones.... But efficient communication requires not only that the right signals are sent: it also requires that those signals are received in a proper way and lead to the right type of action. The cell is enveloped in a thin membrane, which effectively separates the cell's inside from its surroundings. Nonetheless, a chemical signal that reaches the outside of the cell can evoke changes in its inner machinery, changes suited to the needs of the cell and of the entire organism. Alfred G. Gilman and Martin Rodbell have studied this particular aspect of the communication problem.... Among other things, Gilman showed that G proteins work like a timed switch that allows the signal to go through just long enough. G proteins might perhaps be compared to those little gadgets that can

be plugged into a telephone and that make it possible—with a phone call—to turn lamps on and off, start electric heaters, or draw curtains, depending entirely on what the gadget is connected to.[15]

Gilman shaped what is to this day considered to be the premier Department of Pharmacology in the U.S. In 1986 he was the seventh Southwestern faculty member to be elected to the National Academy and in 1994 he became its fourth Nobel laureate, a distinction that as mentioned earlier, is shared by only one other medical school in the world. Parenthetically, Gilman is one of three Nobel laureates who conducted research in Western Reserve's Department of Pharmacology, the others being 1998 Nobel laureate Ferid Murad and 1971 Nobel laureate Earl W. Sutherland, Jr. In addition to the Nobel Prize, Gilman has received the Gairdner Foundation International Award (1984), the Richard Lounsbery Award from the National Academy of Sciences (1987), the Association of American Medical Colleges Award for Distinguished Research in the Biomedical Sciences (1988), the Albert Lasker Basic Medical Research Award (1989), the Louisa Gross Horwitz Prize (Columbia University, 1989), the Passano Foundation Award (1990), the American Heart Association Basic Science Research Prize (1990), the Louis S. Goodman and Alfred Gilman Award in Drug Receptor Pharmacology (American Society of Pharmacology & Experimental Therapeutics, 1990), the Waterford Award (Research Institute of Scripps Clinic, 1990), and the Steven C. Beering Award (Indiana University School of Medicine, 1990). He was elected to membership in the American Academy of Arts & Sciences in 1988 and the Institute of Medicine of the National Academy of Sciences in 1989, and has received honorary degrees from the University of Chicago, Case Western Reserve University, Yale University, and the University of Miami. In 2005, Gilman was appointed the thirteenth Dean of the School of Medicine at UT Southwestern and a year later was designated as Provost of the University and Executive Vice President for Academic Affairs.

※ ※ ※ ※ ※

This chapter began with Charles Cameron Sprague, the medical center's first president. Sprague passed away on September 17, 2005. This milk-drinking boy from Texas made legendary contributions to the growth and maturation of UT Southwestern Medical Center. As Paul M. Bass, chairman of the Southwestern Medical Foundation noted, "Charlie Sprague was the catalyst that enabled UT Southwestern Medical School to grow from a small, relatively unknown institution into one of the most highly respected medical schools in the nation. His unselfish commitment to the medical community and to the well-being of his fellow citizens is unsurpassed." To honor his contributions, the Charles Cameron Sprague Distinguished Chair in Biomedical Science and the Charles Cameron Sprague, MD, Chair in Medical Science were established in 1982 and 1988 respectively, and a new UT Southwestern facility, the Charles Cameron Sprague Clinical Science Building, was named in 1989.

CHAPTER 7

The First Nobel Laureates

The award of the 1985 Nobel Prize in Medicine or Physiology to Joe Goldstein and Mike Brown was arguably the most significant turning point in the history of Southwestern Medical School, instantly and unequivocally transforming its status from very good, or even excellent, to world class. An amusing story involving two of Dallas's great civic leaders, Ralph Rogers and Ross Perot, exemplifies that transformation. (The Dallas community and its civic leadership and philanthropy played critical roles in Southwestern's rise from rags to riches. These are recounted in more detail in chapter 10.)

Ralph B. Rogers was born and raised in Boston. The industrialist and later CEO of Public Broadcasting Service came to Dallas in 1950 to join a company called Texas Industries (not to be confused with another Dallas company, Texas Instruments.) Rogers promoted numerous educational and cultural causes in the city. He had a special interest in medicine and medical research, perhaps stemming from his battle with a severe bout of rheumatic fever as a young man, and served as president of the Dallas Foundation for Health Education and Research. He became well acquainted with the affairs of Southwestern Medical School and Parkland Hospital, and at Charlie Sprague's urging served on the board of managers of the Dallas County Hospital District in the late 1970s, a time of financial crisis for the hospital. Under Rogers' guidance the board orchestrated an $80 million bond issue that reinvigorated Parkland Hospital. He later assisted Sprague with various university projects, including fundraising for the new Zale Lipshy University Hospital that opened in 1990. To show its gratitude, UT Southwestern named the Mary Nell and Ralph B. Rogers Magnetic Resonance Center at Southwestern Medical Center after Rogers and his wife. Rogers was a good friend of Ross Perot, another prominent Dallas businessman. The two were North Dallas neighbors and often chatted when Rogers was out walking and Perot was riding his horses. In his autobiography entitled *Splendid Torch*, Rogers relates the following.

> One morning I went to Ross's office and asked him for a considerable amount of money to enable the University of Texas Southwestern

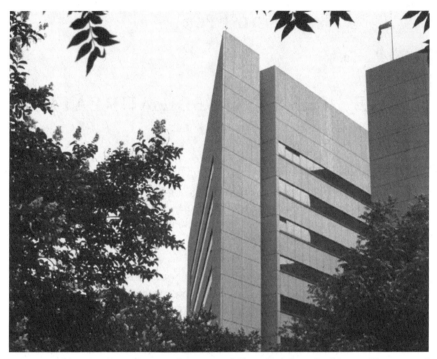

A new Parkland Hospital opened in 1994 following a bond of $80 million voted by Dallas County.

Medical School to take on two important research projects. I had by this time concluded my stint as chairman of the board of Parkland Memorial Hospital and was helping Dr. Charles C. Sprague, President of Southwestern, in his never ceasing effort to make the medical school world class.

I anticipated no great difficulty from Ross because he was always interested in institutions or projects that were 'world class.' Consequently, I put great emphasis on the progress that had been made with the medical school. At the conclusion of my presentation, Ross said that he appreciated the information, but he was not going to comply with my request for a donation. When I expressed some surprise, he said 'You say that Southwestern Medical School is 'world class,' but I have never read about it in the *New York Times*, *Time* magazine, or any of the leading periodicals or newspapers.' I replied that Southwestern Medical School had neither sought, nor worked toward getting publicity, but I was sure that if he inquired among either other leading medical schools or leading doctors or scientists in the field of medicine, they would substantiate my claim that Southwestern was entitled to "world class" designation.

I will never forget Ross's answer. He said, 'Ralph, you have got to learn that perception is more important than reality. Southwestern is not *perceived* [my italics] as 'world class' and I will not accede to your request.' I remember my answer. I said, 'I think that reality is more important than perception, but it is your money I am seeking; you have the sole right to say 'yes' or 'no.''

Some months later I awoke to hear on television, and subsequently read on the front page of the *Dallas Morning News*, that doctors Michael Brown and Joseph Goldstein, both professors at the Southwestern Medical School, had been chosen winners of the Nobel Prize in Medicine. At 9 a.m. I was in the office and dialing Ross Perot. He answered the telephone call, roaring with laughter. He said, 'When I walked into the office this morning, I told all of my associates that I would be hearing from Ralph Rogers today. I said that this was going to cost me.' And so it did.—In subsequent years, Ross has donated millions of dollars; I guess an aggregate of $30,000,000 or more, to what is unquestionably a 'world class' medical school.[1]

✳ ✳ ✳ ✳

Joseph (Joe) Leonard Goldstein and Michael (Mike) Stuart Brown were born almost exactly a year apart (Joe on April 18, 1940, and Mike on April 13, 1941), and met when interning together at the Massachusetts General Hospital in 1966–67. Both pursued postdoctoral research training at the NIH, and both were recruited by Seldin to the faculty of the Department of Internal Medicine at UT Southwestern, where they collaborated on the research that won them the Nobel Prize in Medicine or Physiology in 1985. The collaboration matured to a partnership that endures to this day—a partnership that has flourished because the two scientists agreed long ago to alternate seniority in their scientific publications, to speak their minds freely and openly to one another, and to never allow recruitment efforts to disrupt their partnership. The pair frequently presents formal scientific talks in tag-team fashion, each picking up where the other left off. When they delivered their speeches at the Nobel Banquet in December 1985, Brown began with "Joe and I," and Goldstein with "Michael Brown and I."[2]

In 1966, Brown graduated from the University of Pennsylvania Medical School and won an internship at the Massachusetts General Hospital (MGH)

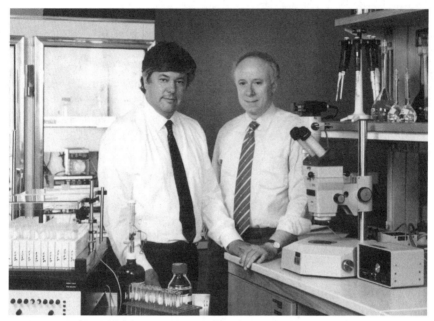

Michael Brown (left) and Joseph Goldstein shown in their laboratory on the day that their Nobel Prize was announced in October 1985.

in Boston (one of the famed teaching hospitals in the Harvard system), a highly coveted beginning to a career in academic medicine. The MGH then admitted only six interns in Internal Medicine each year, and none had hailed from Penn in the past thirteen years. "I was very excited and very proud,"[3] Brown related. "A couple of weeks later I received a list of my fellow interns. I looked down the list and saw the name Goldstein from Southwestern Medical School in Dallas, Texas. I'd never heard of the place, and I thought, 'Oh my God, they must be scraping the bottom of the barrel this year. Probably no one very good applied, so that's why they accepted me—and this jerk from a bible school in Texas!'"[3]

∗ ∗ ∗ ∗ ∗

Born in Brooklyn, Brown grew up in the Philadelphia suburbs. He attended Penn both as an undergraduate and a medical student. From high school on, medical research was his primary ambition.

When I was in high school and wrote the required resume in my college applications I listed a single career goal—medical research. I don't recall being that committed at the time, but obviously I was

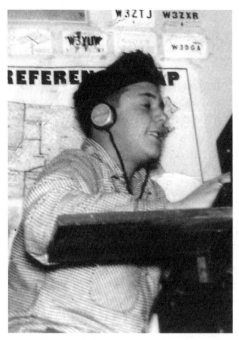

Mike Brown working on his amateur radio transmitter at age 14.

thinking that way. My interest in science came from my amateur radio hobby as a kid. I had a close boyhood friend whose father was an electrical engineer. He interested me in radios, and at age thirteen I had an amateur radio license and built my own transmitters and receivers from plans in magazines. They were pretty complex in those days, and I had to solder a lot of wires. Of course I sometimes made mistakes, and when that happened and I plugged the thing into the wall it blew every fuse in the house. I would then have to meticulously retrace the circuits and do it all over again. In retrospect I think that was a great preparation for doing research. After all, troubleshooting experiments is much of what laboratory research is about.[3]

Brown's father, a textile salesman, hounded him to pursue a career in medicine. "My father always worked for others, and from the time that I was very young he told me that doctors are the only people in the world who are really their own bosses. I'm not sure that he was right, but in the community where I grew up being a doctor was held in high esteem. Both of my parents wanted me to go into medicine, and I'm sure that some of that rubbed off on me."[3] Penn, however, was not Brown's first choice for college.

At high school my self-image was very much that of a pipe-smoking college student. Maybe wearing a scarf or an ascot. Princeton was *the* place in my mind. That was the gentleman's school, and I very much wanted to go there. I was on the waiting list at Princeton when I was informed that I had been admitted to Penn with a full scholarship. A few weeks later I was also admitted to Princeton. But with the scholarship to Penn in hand I could hardly put my parents through the financial burden of Princeton. I was disappointed though—Penn was really way down on my list.[3]

At Penn, the student newspaper occupied much of Brown's attention, almost leading him to a career in journalism.

I have always loved writing, so I joined the student paper, *The Daily Pennsylvanian*. I started out as the sports editor, but later I became the features editor, in charge of the editorial page and the opinions columns. This was the early '60s and the beginning of the counter culture revolution, an exciting and turbulent time if one was involved with a college newspaper. John Kennedy was President and a strong student reaction had emerged against the conservatism of the Eisenhower years. Colleges and universities had been very regimented, with rules for everything. So much so, that in my freshman year a woman wrote a letter to the Philadelphia newspaper complaining that when driving through the Penn campus she had observed students walking around without jackets and ties! So the student newspaper took a very reactionary position. We came out against everything! Against cheerleaders, against fraternities—all that sort of thing. Eventually the university closed our offices down, amid great objection, and we actually went on national television to protest this violation of our freedom of speech.[3]

While at medical school, Brown took a summer research job at Smith Kline Beecham, the large Philadelphia-based pharmaceutical company. During his first summer he was required to measure the effect of various pharmacological compounds on intestinal motility in rats. "The standard method for doing this was to feed the animals charcoal and sacrifice them at various times to determine how far the charcoal had moved through the intestinal tract. I must have sacrificed over ten thousand rats and frankly got quite bored with this. Some of my friends were doing exciting research at the medical school—and here was I pushing charcoal through rats."[3]

Brown's talent for creativity in the laboratory relieved much of the tedium of his required tasks. "I read the scientific literature on the physiology of intestinal motion and began testing all sorts of compounds on my own. Some of them reduced motility; others increased it. Eventually I had enough data to demonstrate that there was a logarithmic decay in intestinal motility as a function of the length of the intestine. In fact I established that the rate of movement of charcoal through the intestine could be predicted mathematically. This saved me a lot of work, because I could predict when to sacrifice many of the rats."[3] Brown published his results, his first scientific publication, in a report called *Intestinal Propulsion in Restrained and Unrestrained Rats*.[4]

While still a medical student, Brown presented the results of these studies at a formal scientific meeting. Several years later, this presentation was pivotal in winning him a research commission at the NIH. Just as his future Southwestern colleagues Jean Wilson and Dan Foster competed for commissions at the NIH during the Korean War, so too did Brown and Goldstein (and Al Gilman) face intense competition during the Vietnam War. "There was no question that I wanted to go to the NIH to do research,"[3] Brown related. "The NIH was a research Mecca then. But getting a position there was extremely competitive."[3]

The NIH awarded research commissions based on a system that attempted to match the interests and expertise of the applicants with its existing research programs. Qualified applicants were required to complete a list that prioritized the research laboratories in which they were most interested. If the head of that laboratory was interested in the applicant, he (or rarely she) might be awarded a coveted commission. To his great relief, Brown found himself matched with a metabolic laboratory.

> There were thirteen laboratories to rank on the form. But at the spur of the moment I decided to pencil in a fourteenth choice, a metabolic laboratory that I was especially interested in. As it turned out I didn't get any of my first thirteen choices. Fortunately for me the person who ran the laboratory that was my fourteenth choice had been in the audience when I presented my talk on intestinal motility and had apparently liked the study. So I got into his lab. If I had not taken the initiative of adding that choice in pencil who knows how my life would have turned out?[3]

✳ ✳ ✳ ✳ ✳

Goldstein's odyssey to a coveted internship in Internal Medicine at the MGH was not dissimilar. Goldstein was born and raised in Kingstree, South Carolina, a town of about 5,000 people where his father ran a department store—and where Goldstein acquired his southern drawl. "It was a typical small southern town," he explained. "The railroad from New York to Florida went through it.

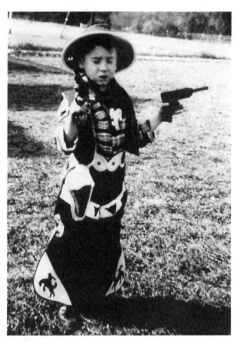

Joe Goldstein at the age of 8—ready to go to Texas!

Blacks lived on one side of the railroad and whites on the other."[5] Like Brown, Goldstein enjoyed a stint as editor of the student newspaper and once interviewed the eighty-five year-old American financier and presidential adviser Bernard Baruch, who owned a winter residence near Kingstree. "I asked him what he advised people like myself to do in the future. He replied that he didn't know much about science; he was a businessman. But he added that science seemed like an important thing to pursue. I put that quote in the student paper."[5] Aside from hearing the great Baruch's inspiring words, Goldstein credits his interest in science to his high school physics and chemistry classes. "In those days teaching in small schools was really good. It was mainly done by well trained teachers, most of whom were women, and they gave one a very well grounded education."[5] Goldstein was president of his high school class and of the student body, and class valedictorian.

Goldstein attended college at Washington and Lee University in Lexington, Virginia, where he majored in chemistry. He planned to complete medical school at Washington University in St. Louis. No sooner had he received formal acceptance, however, than his Texas-born fraternity brothers began extolling the virtues of the medical school in Dallas. "I once casually mentioned this to one of my cousins, an internist," Goldstein stated. "As it happened, he had just returned from a medical meeting and he related to me how much he had enjoyed listening to presentations from Morris Ziff and Don Seldin, two Southwestern faculty members. I was sufficiently impressed that I decided to switch to Southwestern, especially since some of my friends were going there and I really didn't know anyone in St Louis."[5] How different the fates of both UT Southwestern and Washington University School of Medicine might have been had Goldstein stuck with his original intention. [Not that the reader need lament the fate of Washington University, which is widely considered to have one of the premier medical schools in the U.S. Seventeen Nobel laureates have been on its faculty at one time or another.]

Goldstein began medical school in 1962, a time when the Department of Internal Medicine at Southwestern was blossoming. Besides Seldin, the faculty included Dan Foster, Roger Unger, Floyd Rector, Norman Carter, Dennis McGarry, Burton Combes, Jean Wilson, Marvin Siperstein, Morris Ziff, John Fordtran, Norman Kaplan, Carlton Chapman, Jere Mitchell, and John Dietschy. "Within two or three months of the first year the faculty began talking to students about opportunities for research," Goldstein related. "I initially decided that I would work with the head of neurosurgery because I was impressed with his anatomy lectures."[5] But Goldstein's formidable intellect had drawn attention in other quarters, and he was quickly persuaded to spend the next three summers working in the Department of Internal Medicine.

Goldstein was by far the top student in his class. According to Brown, Goldstein's classmates even petitioned the dean to have his test results scored separately because of how badly he skewed the grading curve! His mentors called him "superb" and "something special." In later years, Dan Foster and Jean Wilson wrote: "Joe hit the school like a cyclone and impressed the faculty and the student body as an intellectual dynamo unlike any other student that most of us had ever encountered."[6]

Despite having come from an unknown medical school in "the bible belt," Goldstein made an impression on Brown within a week of beginning his internship. "It was obvious that this fellow Goldstein knew more than anyone else in the group. He knew more than the senior residents. He clearly *was* something special."[3] No intellectual slouch in his own right, Brown was thankful that he had come to Southwestern a year earlier—he'd been able to establish his research laboratory and his reputation independent of Goldstein.

Seldin kept a watchful eye on Goldstein, mentoring him with the intention of later hiring him as a Southwestern faculty member. He helped Goldstein secure an internship at the MGH, and urged him to pursue research training at the NIH. Seldin's plan was for Goldstein to then train in medical genetics (an infant science) with Victor McKusick, the authority on genetics at Johns Hopkins University, and establish a Division of Medical Genetics in the Department of Internal Medicine at Southwestern.

✳ ✳ ✳ ✳

During their internships and residencies, Brown and Goldstein forged a close personal and intellectual rapport. "We found that we shared a lot of interests in common and we hit it off very quickly," Brown related. "We were on hospital call every other night and the interns often met in the hospital cafeteria for so-called midnight supper. At these events Joe and I would talk endlessly about the patients we admitted. But we didn't just discuss clinical issues. Our discussions often turned to what possible biological mechanisms might be operating in certain diseases and how these might be studied in the laboratory."[3] The pair also shared a passion for bridge, and competed as a team in tournaments around Boston.

So began one of the most productive and creative scientific partnerships in modern biology. While formal scientific collaborations between colleagues in the same department or school are not uncommon, it is rare that two individuals jointly operate a single laboratory for their entire careers. This is es-

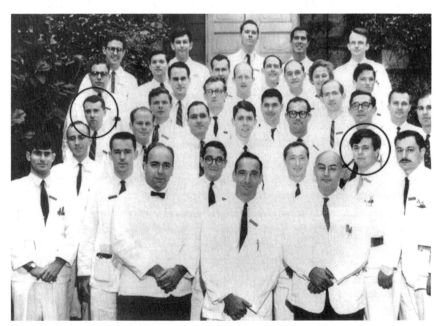

Group photo at the Massachusetts General Hospital in 1967, showing Mike Brown (bottom right) and Joe Goldstein (top left) as residents on the medicine service.

pecially true in the U.S., where the system of reward and promotion encourages the emergence of individual investigators rather than faculty teams.

Having decided that he would return to Southwestern to pursue his academic career, Goldstein began promoting the place to Brown. "Joe kept telling me what a wonderful place Southwestern was. He was tireless in this endeavor. I vividly remember that one night we were on call in the emergency room at the MGH and Joe started in again about Southwestern. We decided to do a comparison between the academic talent at the Mass General and Southwestern. We sat down with a stack of index cards and listed the top people at the MGH in each medical subspecialty. With every name Joe would tell me about equivalent people in Dallas. He hounded me about the place."[3] In due course, Brown heard about the merits of Southwestern from others. "Morris Ziff once came to the MGH as a visiting professor. He was simply mesmerizing. He and his colleagues had just characterized rheumatoid factor and his discussion absolutely fascinated me. On rounds his clinical acumen was impressive too. 'Oh, there are a lot of people like that there,' Joe said nonchalantly. So I began to think seriously about the place."[3]

Goldstein often told Seldin about Brown, how impressive he was. "Don Seldin was a frequent visitor to the northeast, especially around the time of some of the major annual meetings in academic medicine,"[3] Brown related. "During some of these meetings Joe would arrange elaborate dinners for Seldin and invite his fellow residents, including me of course. So I was introduced to Seldin while I was still in training."[3]

Following internship and residency training, Brown and Goldstein departed Boston for the NIH to consummate their research commissions. One year was ostensibly dedicated to clinical duties, the other to laboratory-based research. "The clinical material at the NIH was superb,"[3] Brown related. "The wards were filled with patients with all sorts of rare diseases, including metabolic diseases. As senior residents, we were mainly used as consultants, so there was plenty of time to be in the research laboratory, even during that clinical year."[3]

Brown's experience in the metabolic laboratory to which he was assigned was disappointing. "The laboratory chief was appointed as a scientific adviser to the White House and was away much of the time, and I was left largely to my own devices, unsupervised and undirected. Meanwhile, Joe was in Marshall Nirenberg's lab [Nirenberg was then completing his classic work on the genetic code that would win him a Nobel Prize], and he would come down to my lab and tell me about all the great experiments he was doing. I was pretty miserable for a while."[3] (How remarkable that three of UT Southwestern's Nobel laureates trained at the NIH at the same time.)

Brown was determined to obtain training in classical biochemistry, in particular enzymology (the study of enzymes). With his mentor so often away, however, no one could provide him with the appropriate guidance. Goldstein urged him to switch laboratories, and eventually Brown transferred to one run by Earl Stadtman, a renowned biochemist and enzymologist. "This was one of the most incredible experiences in my life,"[3] Brown related. "For the first time I could work with pure enzymes and do clean experiments that gave clean answers. I was ecstatic!"[3]

Brown was studying a bacterial enzyme called glutamine synthase, and uncovered important aspects of how the enzyme activity is regulated. Indeed, his research assumed such importance to him that he delayed his departure from the NIH for several months to complete his studies. "We had already given up our house in Bethesda and were ready to leave when I told my wife Alice that I needed to stay longer. The only place to live that we could find near the lab was a little shack with no air conditioning. It was summer and I was literally working twenty-four hours a day and Alice was pretty much stuck in this shack alone. This was the first of many occasions when she, without any complaint at all, supported me in what I wanted to do. She was absolutely terrific."[3]

During his initial frustrating laboratory experience, Brown co-authored a series of review articles on gastro-intestinal physiology that were published in the prestigious *New England Journal of Medicine*. In the course of his reading, he encountered the work of the gastroenterology group in the Department of Internal Medicine at Southwestern, further validating Goldstein's high opinion of the place. "I became a genuine admirer of the GI unit. John Fordtran had worked out a lot of the principles of electrolyte and nutrient absorption in the intestine in humans. It was beautiful work. I also read about the work of John Dietschy and Jean Wilson on cholesterol absorption."[3] Eventually, Brown visited Southwestern. "I talked with Seldin and met everyone in the department and I was deeply impressed. I was offered a position as Instructor in the Department of Internal Medicine and immediately accepted it."[3]

As is the rule in American academia, Goldstein and Brown planned to establish independent research laboratories in Dallas. While still at the NIH, however, they decided to work collaboratively on a particular project.

When Joe was on his clinical rotation at the NIH he was looking after two children aged six and eight with the rare homozygous form of familial hypercholesterolemia (FH). [FH occurs in two genetic states. In the homozygous form of the disease, patients are defective in both copies of a particular gene. These individuals have markedly elevated levels of cholesterol in the blood and are typically symptomatic. The heterozygous form of the disease is characterized by a defect in only one of the two relevant genes. Patients have much lower levels of cholesterol and are typically asymptomatic.] Both kids had cholesterol levels of over 1000 (way over the normal levels) and had even suffered myocardial infarcts (heart attacks) as children. They had such bad angina (chest pain from cardiac insufficiency) they couldn't even walk across a room. One day Joe brought me to the ward to see these patients and we began to talk about how we might investigate FH. Joe had been exposed to cholesterol metabolism when he was a medical student through Marvin Siperstein. He knew that Siperstein had determined that an enzyme called 3-hydroxy-3-methylglutaryl coenzyme A reductase (HMG-CoA reductase) was rate-limiting for cholesterol biosynthesis. With my background in enzyme regulation gained in Stadtman's laboratory I was extremely interested in studying this enzyme. Long before we came to Dallas, Joe and I speculated that HMG-CoA reductase might be regulated by binding cholesterol in a particular way and that people with FH have a genetic defect such that their HMG-CoA reductase cannot bind the enzyme properly and thus turn it off. Consequently they over-produce cholesterol. The plan was that when we went to Dallas we'd collaborate on this cholesterol problem and test our hypothesis.[3]

* * * * *

Brown arrived at Southwestern in the fall of 1971. Goldstein would not arrive for another few years. While this first year afforded Brown the opportunity to showcase his considerable academic prowess, he found the initial months difficult.

> I was working with John Dietschy. Dietschy was an excellent physiologist and he was doing fascinating experiments. He would infuse chylomicrons into the thoracic duct of rats, a technically incredibly difficult procedure. One had to insert a tiny catheter into the equally tiny thoracic duct of a rat and secure it so that when one placed the rat in a restraining cage one could collect the lymphatic fluid. It involved incredibly meticulous surgery. I must have done fifty of these procedures, and maybe five of them worked. But during all this time I wanted to work on enzymes. I kept telling Dietschy, 'John, I really want to work on HMG-CoA reductase.'[3]

Such was the extent of Brown's frustration that by Christmas he went back to the MGH to talk to the head of the Division of Gastroenterology about returning there. "He listened and said, 'Well Mike, we can't do that immediately.

Maybe things will improve in Dallas. But if you're still unhappy by June of next year we'll consider you.' After I got back from that Christmas trip I went to see Seldin and told him that while I liked John Dietschy well enough and admired what he was doing, this simply wasn't what I was interested in. I told him that I really wanted to work on this enzyme HMG-CoA reductase."[3] To Brown's surprise, Seldin was sympathetic and steered him to Marvin Siperstein, the faculty expert in cholesterol metabolism.

Teething episodes notwithstanding, Brown has fond memories of the year before Goldstein's arrival.

> It was an incredibly exciting place, both clinically and experimentally. The entire department occupied only about 15,000 square feet, all built around Seldin's office. But Seldin was never *in* his office. He would hang out in the corridor in front of his office, always talking to people. Everyone was in complete awe of the man. We had a number of formal sub-specialty units at the time; gastroenterology, endocrinology, and so on, each with its titular head. But in reality this was a myth. Seldin ran everything! Somebody was certainly called the Head of the GI Unit, or Head of whatever, but I'm not sure what that meant. Seldin headed it all.[3]

Though formally a clinical fellow training in gastroenterology, Brown was able to spend most of his time in the laboratory.

> The residents would see patients and if there was a problem they couldn't handle or if they felt they needed help, they would simply pop over to the lab and drag Dietschy to see a patient. Of course as a GI fellow I would drag along with him. We were so close to Parkland that the house staff could quickly bounce back and forth. And it was easy to attend on the wards because one could usually make rounds for two hours in the morning and have the rest of the day in the lab. The other thing that was incredibly important and stimulating then was that the only convenient place to eat was the hospital cafeteria. So at noon virtually the entire internal medicine faculty and resident staff would gather there. We would sit together and talk well past lunch. It was a very exciting time.[3]

✳ ✳ ✳ ✳ ✳

After completing his research training at the NIH, Goldstein set about becoming a medical geneticist—but not in Baltimore with Victor McKusick as Seldin had planned. Instead, he unilaterally elected to join Arno Motulsky's unit at the University of Washington in Seattle. "In discussing my plans with various people at the NIH I came to realize that McKusick was mainly doing classical human genetics. But having been trained as a biochemist I wanted to apply my biochemical skills to modern human genetics. I heard about Motulsky's program and I met a few people who had worked with him. They gave him rave reviews. So I decided to go to Seattle instead. When I told Seldin he reluctantly said it was all right, but I gather that McKusick was rather disappointed."[5]

In Seattle, Motulsky asked Goldstein what sort of research problem he wanted to pursue. "That was typical of him," Goldstein said. "He would give you the freedom to work on anything you wanted to, and if he liked what you were doing he would give you unlimited support."[5] Goldstein explained his interest in patients with familial hypercholesterolemia without revealing the specific hypothesis that he and Brown planned to test at Southwestern. "This was all much too soft boiled and theoretical to discuss in public then. But we talked about the genetics of familial hypercholesterolemia and we speculated as to whether some people who suffered heart attacks at a young age—before age sixty—might have the heterozygous form of familial hypercholesterolemia (FH)."[5] Not much was known about the heterozygous state of the disease, and Goldstein became interested in determining the true incidence of the condition and whether or not such individuals were predisposed to heart disease. "No one had done a good study to determine what the frequency of elevated cholesterol in the general population was and whether or not this correlated with the risk of heart attacks. So we decided to do a population study. We called it the Seattle Study."[5]

The Seattle Study is now considered a classic in medical genetics. Goldstein and Motulsky assembled a team of nurses, social workers, and computer scientists, and systematically studied 500 survivors of myocardial infarction under the age of sixty. When their analysis was completed, they could confidently report that twenty percent of people who had suffered a heart attack under the age of sixty had elevated cholesterol or triglycerol levels that were determined by one of several genes. The gene causing heterozygous FH was one; it alone could account for as much as five percent of heart attacks in Americans under the age of sixty. FH was now recognized as an important public health problem. Goldstein was also able to deduce that one in 500 people were heterozygous for FH, making the disease one of the most common known inherited genetic diseases. (The severe homozygous form of FH is rarer, occurring with an incidence of about one in a million.) His results were published in the *Journal of Clinical Investigation* in a series of three papers that earned him considerable visibility. By the time he returned to Dallas in 1973, Goldstein had secured a national reputation in the genetics of metabolic diseases.

During his two year sojourn at the University of Washington, Goldstein found time to dabble in Stanley Gartler's laboratory, where Gartler was doing pioneering work in somatic cell genetics. Here, Goldstein learned how to grow cells in tissue culture after procuring them from patients by skin biopsy, a technique that would soon prove crucial for deciphering the fundamental defect in FH.

✳ ✳ ✳ ✳ ✳

Meanwhile, back in Texas, Brown was having difficulty obtaining the purified enzyme he needed in order to study the enzyme HMG-CoA reductase.

> Nobody had successfully purified the enzyme. It was a terrible problem. The enzyme was bound in the endoplasmic reticulum [an intricate network of membranes in living cells] and one of the greatest cholesterol biochemists of all time, Feodor Lynen, who discovered the enzyme activity (and won the Nobel Prize in Medicine or Physiology in 1964) had tried for five years to purify it and was unable to. Lynen wrote in a review article that the enzyme was an intrinsic property of the endoplasmic reticulum and that as soon as it was solubilized it lost activity. So he basically spread the word that it was impossible to purify the enzyme in a water-soluble form. Lynen was Earl Stadtman's great hero. So when just before leaving the NIH when I defiantly told Stadtman that I was going to solubilize and purify HMG-CoA reductase when I got to Dallas, he simply laughed at my bravado![3]

Luck and serendipity play huge roles in science, but it's not pure coincidence that these so-called chance elements often favor the prepared mind. The details of how Brown solved the problem of the insolubility of HMG-CoA reductase in aqueous solutions need not be explained here. It suffices to say that he did so in a fairly short period of time. His paper was published in the *Journal of Biological Chemistry* in 1973. "Aside from the scientific importance of this breakthrough, this was a very significant psychological breakthrough for me, because it happened before Joe arrived in Dallas. If Joe had already been here you could imagine how this work might have been received."[3] Years later, the enzyme HMG-CoA reductase became the successful target of a class of cholesterol-reducing drugs called statins, now multi-billion dollar pharmacological agents that have saved countless people from heart disease.

With Goldstein and Brown united once again, the pair settled into their new roles as faculty members. Both had clinical responsibilities (which Seldin required of his entire faculty), Brown as a gastroenterologist and Goldstein as a medical geneticist. Both quickly acquired NIH grant support to operate research projects in their respective laboratories. But most importantly, they began testing the hypothesis that they had formulated while at the NIH. Within a few years, their collaborative research became so productive that they dropped their other research efforts to pursue this investigation exclusively. "I had an NIH grant to study something else. But when I informed them of the exciting stuff going on with the FH studies they allowed me to switch my grant support with no fuss,"[5] Goldstein related.

✳ ✳ ✳ ✳ ✳

Brown and Goldstein desperately sought access to patients with the homozygous form of FH, the full-blown state of the disease in which blood cholesterol levels can be enormously increased and death from a heart attack is a near certainty. In particular, they wanted a skin biopsy from a patient so that they could grow and study living cells. Goldstein had educated himself on the novel techniques of growing and propagating human cells in tissue culture while he was at the University of Washington, precisely in order to conduct such studies. Gaining access to patients with the homozygous state of FH, let alone acquiring skin biopsies, was not a trivial matter. The homozygous state of the disease is rare, and most cases ended up in specialized research centers such as the NIH. The children that Brown and Goldstein had observed while research fellows at the NIH "belonged" to Donald Fredrickson, later director of the NIH, who was studying FH with his own research team. Brown and Goldstein, therefore, searched for other cases.

Their opportunity providentially arrived in 1973 when a pediatrician contacted Marvin Siperstein's office about a hospitalized case of FH in Denver, Colorado. As Siperstein was on sabbatical in Switzerland, his secretary thankfully asked the pediatrician if he would like to speak with Siperstein's young associate, Michael Brown. As it turned out, the pediatrician had been at the NIH at the same time as Brown. Brown explains what the pediatrician told him that day.

He told me this fantastic story. They had a twelve year old child with FH with a serum cholesterol of over 1000. She could hardly walk across the room and was dying. Tom Starzl [a renowned organ transplant surgeon at the University of Colorado] was going to perform a desperate novel surgical procedure on her in the next few days and he wanted Siperstein to fly to Denver to obtain a liver biopsy to measure cholesterol levels in the liver. I was stunned. I said, 'Well you realize that we don't have any controls. I have no idea what the normal rate of cholesterol synthesis in the liver is. In addition, this patient has been in the hospital on a special diet and she'll be under anesthesia. We'll have no real idea how to interpret the results.' But my colleague remonstrated that he was simply acting on the instructions of Starzl, who wanted this done. So I said, 'OK, I'll come up. But in exchange I want a little piece of skin from the surgical incision.'[3]

Brown flew to Denver, ostensibly to promote Starzl's research program, but in fact to acquire the precious skin biopsy—with no collaborative strings attached. "I carried this huge bag of stuff with me because Jean Wilson admonished me that even though I was going to a university, I shouldn't assume that they would have everything there that I would need."[3] Brown brought the skin biopsy back to Dallas, where Goldstein prepared it for tissue culture. The ensuing weeks, while the cells were growing, were nerve-wracking—much could go wrong in those pioneering days, including the complete failure of the cells to grow. Finally, the cells were successfully cultured and harvested and ready to be tested. Goldstein explains what they found.

The first results were simply incredible. They were so clear-cut it was almost unbelievable. We knew from our previous work that if one grew normal human cells in the presence of fetal calf serum so that the cells didn't have to synthesize their own cholesterol, cholesterol synthesis in the cells was low. But if one removed the fetal calf serum, the cells upregulated their cholesterol biosynthesis. We also knew that in normal cells cholesterol synthesis and HMG-CoA reductase are inhibited by low-density lipoprotein (LDL). But in these FH cells the cholesterol synthesis was about 100 times higher than normal, even in the presence of fetal calf serum. Furthermore, the enzyme HMG-CoA reductase was totally unresponsive to added LDL.[5]

Around the time that the cells were ready to be tested, Brown went to a meeting in Atlantic City, which was then a proverbial Mecca for annual biological science meetings.

One evening I returned to my hotel and there was a message from Joe that he was at a dinner party at Don Seldin's home in Dallas and urgently wanted me to call him there. 'You aren't going to believe this,' Joe shouted excitedly over the phone. And he told me the results. I remember running excitedly onto the boardwalk in Atlantic City not knowing exactly what to do next. I encountered a group of friends who were former residents from the MGH and joined them for dinner. During the entire meal I sat there thinking to myself that even

though this was only one experiment, we had stumbled onto something very important.[3]

Indeed they had. While much work remained to be done to obtain a definitive explanation of the genetic defect in FH, the duo had a firm biochemical
handle on the problem. With a little luck, deciphering it would only be a matter of time and hard work.

Brown and Goldstein were eager to publish their initial findings. "But Jean
Wilson and Dan Foster admonished us that we shouldn't publish results from
just a single patient," Goldstein related. "What if this was some sort of fluke
that was somehow unique to that particular patient's cells?"[5] Brown and Goldstein set about locating other patients with the homozygous form of FH, eventually identifying a physician in Canada with two cases.

"Mike and I flew up to Montreal on an Eastern Airlines shuttle from New
York [to obtain skin biopsies]. We were literally on pins and needles about our
results and whether they would be reproducible. When we got off the plane
we were utterly startled by dozens of cameras flashing at us. There were pho-
tographers and reporters all over the place and we were presented with red
roses. We thought, 'My God, they must know our secret!' But it turned out
that one of us was the one millionth passenger to have flown this Eastern Airlines shuttle!"[5]

When repeat experiments confirmed their initial findings, Brown and
Goldstein set about systematically dissecting the biochemical and molecular
basis of the hereditary disease FH. As their research progressed, they disproved
their original hypothesis about a defect in HMG-CoA reductase, the rate-limiting enzyme for cholesterol biosynthesis. After several more years, they
demonstrated that individuals with FH are in fact defective in a receptor on
the surface of cells that normally binds low-density lipoproteins (LDL), and
that this defect triggers abnormal cholesterol levels. Suffice it to say that their
discoveries had a staggering impact on our understanding of the regulation of
cholesterol metabolism. In their press release on the occasion of the 1985
Nobel Prize in Medicine or Physiology, the Nobel Foundation stated:

> Michael S. Brown and Joseph L. Goldstein have through their discov-
> eries revolutionized our knowledge about the regulation of cholesterol
> metabolism and the treatment of diseases caused by abnormally ele-
> vated cholesterol levels in the blood. They found that cells on their
> surfaces have receptors which mediate the uptake of the cholesterol-
> containing particles called low-density lipoprotein (LDL) that circu-
> late in the blood stream. Brown and Goldstein have discovered that
> the underlying mechanism of the severe hereditary familial hypercho-

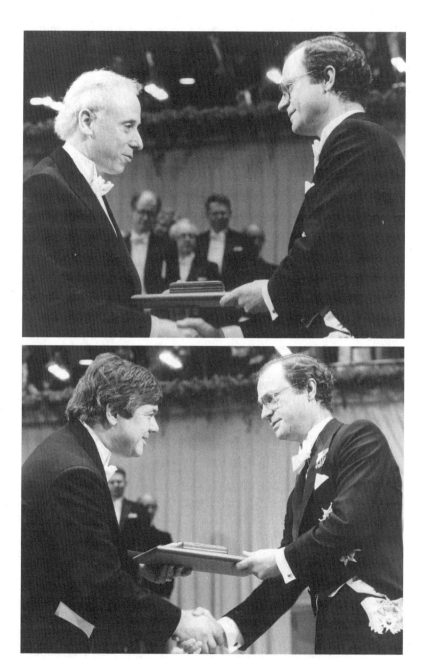

Joe Goldstein (top) and Mike Brown (bottom) receiving the 1985 Nobel Prize in Physiology or Medicine from King Carl XVI Gustaf of Sweden.

lesterolemia is a complete, or partial, lack of functional LDL-receptors. In normal individuals the uptake of dietary cholesterol inhibits the cells own synthesis of cholesterol. As a consequence the number of LDL-receptors on the cell surface is reduced. This leads to increased levels of cholesterol in the blood, which subsequently may accumulate in the wall of arteries causing atherosclerosis and eventually a heart attack or a stroke. Brown and Goldstein's discoveries have lead to new principles for treatment, and prevention, of atherosclerosis.[7]

Beyond the immediate medical implications of their discoveries, Brown and Goldstein's work opened new vistas in cell biology. "Little was known about receptors on cell surfaces," Goldstein stated. "Certainly no one had any idea that proteins could enter cells by binding to receptors and then being internalized into special compartments in cells, a process that we called receptor-mediated endocytosis. This attracted the attention of cell biologists working in diverse systems."[5]

Over the years, Brown and Goldstein, and subsequently other researchers, demonstrated that patients with FH can have varying degrees of hypercholesterolemia ranging from very mild to very severe, depending on the type of mutation in the gene that encodes their LDL receptor. All three of their original cases happened to have mutations that produced no receptors at all, causing a severe "all or none" defect in the tissue culture system. "We could easily have encountered cases with partial defects," Brown recalled. "If we had I believe that we might have dropped the project there and then. We weren't prepared for dealing with the complexities of partial defects then. We both had other projects going on in our labs, and I really think that we would have dropped the FH story."[3]

✻ ✻ ✻ ✻ ✻

Brown and Goldstein have often been asked what stresses have affected their relationship. Brown explains how they were able to make the collaboration work.

I think we probably have the longest scientific collaboration in American science, other than the Coris,' [Carl and Gerty Cori were a famous husband and wife team of biochemists who won the Nobel Prize for Physiology or Medicine in 1947], and *they* were married to each other. In many ways our relationship has been very much like a marriage—in the sense that it's been something that we have had to work at all the time. From the very beginning of our success we discussed this. As individuals we had both enjoyed our fair share of achieving scientific excellence—and of getting credit for it individually. Now suddenly we were in this sharing mode. So we made a solemn pact that neither of us would ever take sole credit for ideas that came out of our collaboration. We both fully recognized that if I happened to say something interesting on Wednesday, it was probably because Joe had said something that planted an idea in my mind on Monday, and vice versa. So to say, 'This was *my* idea, or this was *your* idea,' would have been an absolute disaster. For years we have strictly rotated first authorship and last authorship on our publications, and we operate all aspects of our research laboratory jointly.[3]

"The biggest challenge to establishing a long-term collaboration is to get into the habit of thinking aloud," Goldstein once stated. "When you think alone, you have the luxury of coming up with lousy ideas and secretly rejecting them. But with a collaborator, you have to overcome the embarrassment of sharing each other's lunacy. Once two collaborators become accustomed to thinking aloud, the constant dialogue creates a remarkable energy and synergy of the minds, often propelling the research into unforeseen directions."[6]

Brown makes no pretensions about the challenges of such long-term collaborations.

I strongly believe that a collaboration like ours requires that one of the parties, and *only* one, be a saint. Because if both of you are saints everybody's going to be too nice to one another and nothing will get done. And if neither is a saint there will be so much arguing that again nothing will get done. I'm not the saint. But Joe has the extraordinary ability to handle the pressure when things aren't working, or when we seriously disagree. And we have had plenty of disagreements. But we never disagree about fundamental issues. We may disagree as to whether to do an experiment with a low magnesium concentration or a high magnesium concentration sort of thing, but when it comes to the major directions that we're going to take—the major next problem to tackle, we never disagree. All of this is based on strong mutual respect. We respect one another's opinions, and, as it happens, we like one another.[3]

✳ ✳ ✳ ✳ ✳

Before long, other institutions began trying to recruit Brown and Goldstein. The two never seriously considered any of the offers, resisting even Harvard, the Rockefeller Institute, and Stanford. "Of course some of these offers were flattering," Goldstein commented. "But we were very involved with our research. Starting with the mid- and late-1970s and into the early 1980s, we always had important experiments to do and important papers to write, and in the main we found these offers distracting."[5]

They did give serious thought to one offer. In the late 1970s, the Gladstone Foundation, founded by the shopping center magnate J. David Gladstone, decided to build an institute in San Francisco dedicated to the study of heart disease—and wanted Brown and Goldstein at the helm.* Brown and Goldstein related what transpired.

> They had a lot of space and a lot of money, and we were very sorely tempted. But Southwestern went to tremendous efforts to keep us here. We were rapidly promoted and they established a new Department of Molecular Genetics with one of us (Joe Goldstein) as chairman, and a new Center with the other (Mike Brown) as the Center Director. The reality is that at Southwestern we had everything we needed, which, in those early days before gene cloning, was not much more than some fibroblasts, a few biochemical assays, and our collective brains! And we were so excited about our work that we didn't really want to suffer the delays of setting up a new laboratory. We recognized early on that we needed to collaborate with a cell biologist who knew something about lysosomes. But we had Dick Anderson right here. [Richard Anderson, a prominent cell biologist, is presently chairman of the Department of Cell Biology at UT Southwestern.][3,5]

Sprague and Seldin did everything they could to keep Brown and Goldstein secure in Dallas. Goldstein explains how Sprague was instrumental to their winning a research grant from the NIH.

> By this time our former competitor, Don Fredrickson, was Director of the NIH, and was very gracious and complimentary about our work. Charlie Sprague was on one of Fredrickson's advisory councils and explored with him if there was any way that we could apply for a program project grant to support our work. This was in 1976 and we had just begun to collaborate with Dick Anderson, who was then a new faculty member in the Department of Cell Biology. When we applied for the grant there were just the three of us, Mike, Dick and me. I think it established a record for the smallest number of investigators on a program project grant.[5]

---

* Parenthetically, it's remarkable to note that the Gladstone Institute of Cardiovascular Disease is presently directed by a highly accomplished former UT Southwestern faculty member, Deepak Srivastava, now the Wilma and Adeline Pirag Distinguished Professor in Pediatric Developmental Cardiology at the University of California, San Francisco.

At the time of this writing, Brown and Goldstein's program project grant (now in its twenty-ninth year) had grown to nine investigators. It remains their only formal source of grant funding.

* * * * *

Beginning in 1974 with the Heinrich Wieland Prize for Research in Lipid Metabolism, accolades for Brown and Goldstein (and for UT Southwestern) poured in. The couple shared the Pfizer Award for Enzyme Chemistry of the American Chemical Society (1976), the Albion O. Bernstein Award of the New York State Medical Society (1977), the Passano Award (1978), the Lounsbery Award of the U.S. National Academy of Sciences (1979), the Gairdner Foundation International Award and the New York Academy of Sciences Award in Biological and Medical Sciences (1981), and the Lita Annenberg Hazen Award (1982). By 1984, when Brown and Goldstein were recognized with the V. D. Mattia Award of the Roche Institute of Molecular Biology, the Distinguished Research Award of the Association of American Medical Colleges, the Research Achievement Award of the American Heart Association, and the Louisa Gross Horwitz Award of Columbia University, the Nobel Prize was on everyone's lips. The following year brought the 3M Life Sciences Award of the Federation of American Societies for Experimental Biology, the William Allan Award of the American Society of Human Genetics, and the Albert D. Lasker Award in Basic Medical Research (the so-called American Nobel). Finally, in October 1985, the early morning phone call came from Stockholm informing them that they had been awarded the Nobel Prize in Medicine or Physiology.

Ross Perot was not the only one to question the world-class status of the University of Texas Health Sciences Center at Dallas. Soon after the award of the 1985 Nobel Prize in Medicine or Physiology to Brown and Goldstein was announced, the late Sir John Maddox, for many years the august editor of *Nature*, wrote an editorial piece in the journal stating: "So far all attempts to lure both of them from their opulent Dallas surroundings to more distinguished institutions have failed."[8] This prompted New York University rheumatologist Gerald Weissmann to rush to the defense of the Dallas institution with the following rejoinder: "As a longtime admirer not only of our new laureates but of the remarkable medical school in which they work, permit me to suggest that it might be hard, indeed, to identify 'more distinguished institutions.' Considering the high level of innovative science that is conducted at the University of Texas Health Sciences Center at Dallas, I look forward to Newmark's revised estimate of Dallas as more of her sons share the dais with the King of Sweden."[9] Weissmann must have taken great personal pleasure when in the course of the next decade two more of UT Southwestern's sons did indeed share the dais with the King of Sweden.

In closing this brief discourse on Nobel Prizes and their recognition, it is appropriate to mention that one of the co-recipients of the 2004 Nobel Prize in Physiology or Medicine, Linda Buck, PhD, was mentored as a graduate student at UT Southwestern by Dr. Ellen Vitteta in the Department of Microbiology. The university celebrated the success of one of its graduate students with the same pride and pleasure that it did the four faculty laureates.

CHAPTER 8

EXPANDING IN DIFFICULT TIMES — THE WILDENTHAL YEARS

Between the mid-1960s and the mid-1980s, UT Southwestern and other Texas institutions of higher learning were generously endowed with state and federal funds. In 1965 the state budget appropriation for the medical school was $2.5 million. By 1985, this figure had risen to a whopping $62.5 million. Just one year later, however, a sudden drop in the price of oil caused the state's economy to fall into recession and the real estate and banking markets to collapse. The days of essentially unlimited state support were over!

Kern Wildenthal, Sprague's successor as president of the medical center in 1986, had barely managed to reorganize his desk when he was told that his fiscal year 1986–87 budget would be cut by ten percent. "This news came with the solemn warning that the decreased budget level would be perpetuated until further notice," Wildenthal commented. "We were suddenly thrown into a serious financial crisis—at a time when we were fundamentally poised to move forward and capitalize on the huge gains made over the past few decades."[1]

✳ ✳ ✳ ✳ ✳

When he graduated from UT Southwestern medical school in 1964, Wildenthal had no intention of becoming president of this or any other medical school. Born and raised in Texas, Wildenthal was another addition to Seldin's physician-scholar faculty, and sought a career in academic cardiology. "After completing residency and fellowship training in cardiology I wanted to pursue research involving tissue and organ culture. One of my mentors at the National Heart Institute told me about a leading figure in organ culture at Cambridge University and advised me to consider working with her."[1]

Wildenthal acquired his PhD at Cambridge, England, and stayed on for postdoctoral work before returning to Southwestern in 1970 as an assistant professor in the Departments of Internal Medicine and Physiology. His an-

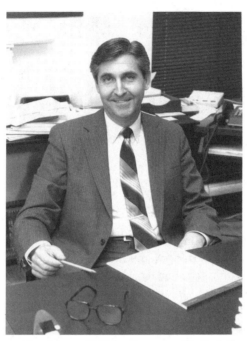

Kern Wildenthal served as Dean of UT Southwestern Medical Center from 1980–86 and has been president of the organization since 1986.

ticipated career began promisingly. "I obtained research grants and was publishing independently, and I was promoted to associate professor after my second year on the faculty."[1] Wildenthal quickly rose through the academic ranks, and in 1975 obtained a Guggenheim Fellowship to pursue a year of further research abroad. "I returned to Cambridge to work with a different person in a new area of research," he related. "But I was able to keep my laboratory at Southwestern going by long distance."[1]

By the early 1970s, the graduate school at Southwestern had matured to the point that it required a dedicated dean, though initially only on a part-time basis. Ron Estabrook, Chairman of the Department of Biochemistry, assumed the task. In due course, however, he resigned in order to devote more attention to both the biochemistry department and his own research program. A national search identified a new dean, but the individual precipitously withdrew from the appointment a few days before the start of the 1976–77 academic year. "Almost as soon as I returned from Cambridge Charlie Sprague summoned me to his office and informed me that he wanted me to take on the duties of acting dean," Wildenthal related. "I thought about this and eventually decided that I could manage this responsibility without relinquishing my academic activities. So I told Sprague that I was willing to serve as acting dean of the graduate school—with the condition that I not be considered for the permanent position."[1] Though determined to pursue a career in academic medicine, Wildenthal had not ruled out an eventual administrative leadership role. "I thought that if I continued to be successful with my research I might eventually become head of a cardiology division somewhere, or even head of a department of internal medicine, or a department of physiology. So when Sprague approached me to be acting dean of the graduate school I thought that it might be interesting to have a part time administrative job that could teach me more about the inner workings of a medical school."[1]

Little did Wildenthal realize that his part-time position as acting dean would mark the beginning of a career in academic administration. Within six months, the search committee urged him to offer his candidacy for the position of permanent dean of the graduate school. He agreed. "By then I really liked this new role. I had determined that it could be done without interfering with my academic activities or research. In fact I had acquired more research grants. I enjoyed being involved with the students and I also liked the involvement with the affairs of the school."[1] When a formal offer came soon after, Wildenthal accepted.

"I settled in as graduate school dean from 1976 to 1980 and discovered during that period that I had a knack for and enjoyed administration."[1] Even though his arena of responsibility was ostensibly confined to the graduate school, Wildenthal was involved in broader medical center issues. "We were still a pretty small institution and basically all issues were analyzed by just four of us. Besides Charlie Sprague, Fred Bonte, Julius Weeks (the Vice-President for Business Affairs) and I were it! We all sat at the same table making decisions, and while I personally didn't have that much authority, I came to understand the institution very well. I also had occasion to meet often with the chairs of both the basic science and clinical departments, and faced the many challenges of co-coordinating department chairs among themselves and with the central administration."[1]

By 1979, word of Wildenthal's administrative skills had spread. He was invited to explore both the chairmanship of the Department of Physiology at Baylor Medical College in Houston, and the deanship of the medical school at the University of Nebraska. "I quickly decided against Nebraska. But the opportunity to build physiology at Baylor was attractive and I thought about it a lot."[1] But by this time Wildenthal had acquired a taste and aptitude for central administration. Moreover, the Nebraska offer led him to believe that he might some day be considered for such a position elsewhere. He declined the offer. "I decided that I enjoyed central administration more than administering a department."[1]

Wildenthal was then indeed on the short list of medical school dean candidates at other institutions, and a short few months later he declined an offer from the University of California at Davis. But in early 1980, Baylor Medical College came courting again, this time offering the deanship. "When I turned down the physiology chair at Baylor I had told them that I really hoped to be dean of a medical school someday. As it happened, their dean's position fell vacant, and president Bill Butler asked me to come down and look at the position. I was now faced with a tough decision, because I realized that at that point of my career there was not likely to be a better opportunity to be dean of a medical school."[1] Wildenthal was sorely tempted but he felt a strong allegiance to the institution in which he had prospered since his days as a medical student. Fortunately for all (except perhaps Baylor College of Medicine), his dilemma was quickly resolved when Fred Bonte retired and Sprague appointed a search committee that nominated him to be the ninth dean of UT Southwestern Medical School.

✳ ✳ ✳ ✳ ✳

At the start of the 1980s, Southwestern Medical School (known then as the University of Texas Health Sciences Center at Dallas) was a very reputable academic institution. The Department of Internal Medicine was internationally prominent, and the basic science departments of biochemistry, cell biology, microbiology, and physiology were thriving. To add to the existing Cary, Hoblitzelle, and Danciger Buildings, Sprague had erected the Florence Bioinformation Center, the Philip R. Jonsson Basic Science Research Building, the Cecil H. and Ida Green Science Building, the Harry S. Moss Clinical Science Building, the impressive Tom and Lula Gooch Auditorium, and the Eugene McDermott Academic Administration Building, now affectionately referred to as "the tower". "There had been huge improvement and consolidation in the late '60s and throughout the '70s," Wildenthal commented. "Those were fiscally healthy times, and the state was literally pouring money into universities in Texas. State allocations were largely based on student enrollment, and institutions with medical and dental schools did particularly well, especially after class sizes were doubled. Federal funds were also increasing the budget at a steady rate."[1]

Federal and state funding was so stable that Sprague rarely had to approach Dallas community leaders or the Southwestern Medical Foundation for assistance. In fact, he had not actively solicited funds from the foundation since the $7.5 million shortfall experienced during the capital expansion in the early 1970s. Wildenthal explained the school's financial position.

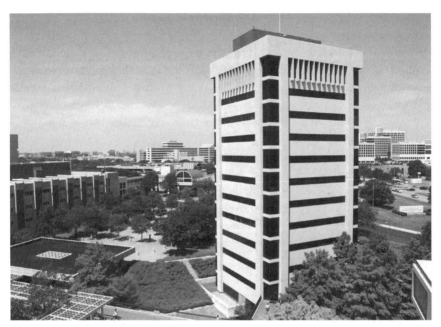

The south campus circa 1990, showing the imposing Eugene McDermott Academic Administration Building in the front center.

For a twenty-year period from the mid-1960s to the mid-1980s it was a lot easier to go to Austin and get your fifteen to twenty percent increase each year. It was generally assumed that these increases would go on forever. Indeed, when I became dean in 1980, we were looking forward to the next big push and there were no conceptual limits to our ambitions. I knew that we needed to rebuild pharmacology, and several other departments. Additionally, the molecular biology revolution was in full swing and we realized that we didn't have much of a formal molecular biology presence at Southwestern. So that had to be put in place as well. In addition, with Children's Medical Center's presence on the campus we recognized major opportunities in pediatrics that would require financial resources. The institution had ambitious plans, and with state resources still growing at that time, we were able to retain our top faculty leaders, attract spectacular new talent, and launch a number of new initiatives that improved the institution immeasurably.[1]

✳ ✳ ✳ ✳ ✳

With Gilman on board to head the Department of Pharmacology, attention shifted to the urgent need for leadership in the rapidly emerging discipline of molecular biology, especially in the exploding arena of gene cloning. Philip Sharp of MIT was identified as a possible new chairman of biochemistry, but negotiations moved slowly. As did Gilman when originally approached by Southwestern, Sharp declined the offer so as not to interrupt his research program at MIT, a strategy that eventually won him a Nobel Prize too.

In 1984, Joe Goldstein was visiting the Cold Spring Harbor Laboratory on Long Island, New York. There he met Joseph (Joe) Sambrook, an internationally recognized molecular virologist whom Cold Spring Harbor Laboratory director James Watson had recruited to spearhead efforts in cancer research. Aside from his important research contributions on tumor viruses, Sambrook and several of his colleagues had recently written a definitive and enormously successful laboratory manual on gene cloning entitled *Molecular Cloning: A Laboratory Manual*. (The "Sambrook manual" is now in its 3rd edition, and every modern biology research laboratory in the world has at least one copy on its shelves.)

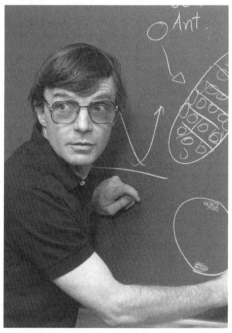

Joseph (Joe) Sambrook, a leading molecular biologist, chaired the Department of Biochemistry from 1986–1992. Sambrook is a Fellow of the Royal Society of London.

"I was telling him about what was going on at Southwestern and informed him that we had offered the chairmanship of biochemistry to Phil Sharp, but that he was probably not going to take it," Goldstein related. "Out of the blue Sambrook asked, 'What about me for the job?' I was quite taken aback. But I replied: 'That's an interesting idea. What *about* you?' "[2] Goldstein returned to Dallas and informed Brown and Gilman of Sambrook's categorical interest.

Few of the senior scientists at Southwestern were optimistic that Sambrook would leave the protected academic environment of the Cold Spring Harbor Laboratory, where he was likely to succeed the venerable James Watson as director. Much to their delight, they were wrong. Sambrook accepted the position of professor and chairman of the Department of Biochemistry. He not only provided the school with instant visibility in cutting edge molecular biology, but, recognizing that structural biology was not represented at UT Southwestern, set about building a world class unit in X-ray crystallography.

An important milestone that coincided with Sambrook's recruitment facilitated much of this new growth and development. In 1985, UT Southwestern was designated a member of the elite Howard Hughes Medical Institute. Howard R. Hughes is remembered by most as an eccentric billionaire who spent the last years of his life in virtual isolation, cultivating impossibly long fingernails. He was, however, a man of extraordinary intellect, energy, and diverse talents. He dabbled in movies; designed, constructed, and raced airplanes; built TWA into a premier international airline; and developed Hughes Aircraft Company into one of the country's largest and most important defense contractors.[3]

His most enduring accomplishment, however, is probably the creation of the Howard Hughes Medical Institute. Hughes's vision of scientific philanthropy was neither modest nor ordinary. He wanted his institute to be committed to basic research, to probe "the genesis of life itself."[3] In 1984, a group of trustees reaffirmed the institute's primary purpose of basic medical research and guided it through the sale of the Hughes Aircraft Company (which the institute owned) and the ensuing period of rapid expansion.[3] The Howard Hughes Medical Institute is now the nation's largest private source of support for biomedical research and science education, making annual contributions approaching $500 million.

In the early 1980s, only a dozen handpicked academic establishments in the U.S. enjoyed membership in the Howard Hughes Institute. The benefits were, and still are, considerable. The institute supports the entire cost, including salaries, of a group of elite hand-picked Howard Hughes Investigators at a designated academic institution, even renting research space or underwriting the construction of new facilities. "They awarded us $7 million a year, which was very substantial money in those days,"[1] Wildenthal commented.

"The timing was perfect," Goldstein related. "Sambrook and his scientist wife Mary Jane Gething came to Dallas with the understanding that Mary Jane would be a Hughes Investigator and Joe, who was ineligible for a Hughes investigatorship by dint of being a department chair, would be in charge of recruiting other investigators to the institute."[2] Armed with several prestigious Howard Hughes Investigatorships, Sambrook went in search of a premier structural biologist and landed Johann (Hans) Deisenhofer, an outstanding X-ray crystallographer from the Max Planck Institute in Munich who had just completed an impressive body of work—one that would win him a Nobel Prize soon after he joined the faculty at UT Southwestern.

✳ ✳ ✳ ✳ ✳

A modest man with a charming manner, Johann Deisenhofer grew up in rural post-war southern Bavaria. His parents were farmers, and expected him to follow in the family tradition. "At that time farming was a sensible and profitable occupation because food was badly needed after the war," Deisenhofer recounted. "But I was not at all interested in farming. Eventually my parents decided that if I wasn't going to be a farmer I should at least obtain a solid education."[4] The rural Bavarian community, however, provided only a rudimentary education, and by the time his parents decided to make serious schooling a priority, Deisenhofer was well behind his peer group. "I had also been pretty lazy at school," Deisenhofer smilingly admitted. "So I had to spend a lot of extra time catching up on subjects like English and Latin."[4] The challenges of a more rigorous education, however, stirred his intellectual prowess, and Deisenhofer persevered, living alone in a strange town to complete high school and gain entrance to the Technical University of Munich. By this time, he had decided to pursue physics as a career. In the course of his formal studies at the Technical University of Munich, he encountered the embryonic field of biophysics, a discipline in which modern physical techniques were applied to biological problems. Excited by this newfound interest, Deisenhofer elected to pursue graduate studies in protein X-ray crystallography at the prestigious Max Planck Institute.

Deisenhofer remained at the Max Planck as a postdoctoral fellow, and in 1976 was appointed a junior member of the scientific staff. In the early 1980s he joined an ambitious project aimed at solving the structure of the photosynthetic reaction center of a bacterium (called *Rhodopseudomonas viridis*). The photosynthetic reaction center is composed of a large protein complex embedded in the cell membrane of the bacterium—a formidable challenge to structural biologists, as no one had managed to purify protein complexes from cell membranes of the quality and quantity required for X-ray crystallographic studies. The success that eventually enjoined this project won Deisenhofer considerable visibility, prompting him to visit several institutions in search of a permanent position that would enable him to direct his own research group. While at the European Molecular Biology Laboratory in Heidelberg, he discussed his ambitions with the former director, John Tooze, who, having heard through the academic grapevine that UT Southwestern was in the market for precisely such an individual, forwarded Deisenhofer's name to Joe Sambrook.

"I received a formal letter from Joe Sambrook (whom I had never heard of) asking whether I might be interested in a faculty position at what was then the University of Texas Health Sciences Center. I knew absolutely nothing about the place, or about Dallas. But a post-doctoral fellow in our research group in Munich had completed his PhD at Baylor College of Medicine in Houston, and spoke highly of UT Southwestern. So I decided to visit the place."[4] Deisenhofer visited Southwestern in 1986, and was immediately impressed with the breadth and depth of the basic sciences. Additionally, he was struck by the collegial, interactive, and forward-looking attitudes, and appreciated the benefits of being a Howard Hughes Investigator. "Sambrook told me about his plan to build structural biology as part of the Hughes Institute. He had already hired Betsy Goldsmith and Steve Sprang, both of whom seemed like wonderful potential colleagues."[4] Deisenhofer agreed to a second visit in early 1987. "I well remember the day that I arrived on my second visit. It was one of those glorious winter days in Texas when the sky is a clear, clear blue and the temperature is in the low 70s. In Munich I had endured three solid weeks of cold, fog and drizzle; so the contrast was very striking!"[4]

During both visits, Sambrook asked a European member of his faculty, Kirsten Fischer-Lindahl, a distinguished immunologist and formerly also a Howard Hughes Investigator, to show Deisenhofer around the city. "Almost immediately after I met her I fell in love with Kirsten,"[4] Deisenhofer smilingly related. Deisenhofer's mind was made up, and he joined the faculty to UT Southwestern in March 1988 as a Hughes Investigator in Sambrook's new Department of Biochemistry. Six months later, he received the coveted early morning phone call from Stockholm informing him that he was a co-recipient of the 1988 Nobel Prize in Chemistry. In his presentation speech at the Nobel ceremonies in December 1988, a member of the Swedish Academy of Sciences stated:

> For a long time it has been impossible to prepare membrane-bound proteins in a form allowing the determination of the detailed structure in three dimensions. Before 1984, there were only rather fuzzy structural pictures available for a few membrane proteins. These had been

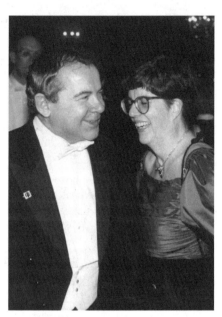

Johann Deisenhofer and his wife, UT Southwestern faculty member Kirsten Fischer-Lindahl, enjoying the 1988 Nobel Prize festivities.

derived with the aid of an electron microscopic method.... But the situation had actually drastically changed in 1982, when Hartmut Michel ... succeeded in preparing highly ordered crystals of a photosynthetic reaction center from a bacterium. With these crystals he could in the period 1982–1985, in collaboration with Johann Deisenhofer and Robert Huber, determine the structure of the reaction center in atomic detail. [This] structural determination ... has led to a giant leap in our understanding of fundamental reactions in photosynthesis, the most important chemical reaction in the biosphere of our earth. But it has also consequences far outside the field of photosynthesis research. Not only photosynthesis and respiration are associated with membrane-bound proteins, but also many other central biological functions, e.g., the transport of nutrients into cells, hormone action or nerve impulses. Proteins participating in these processes must span biological membranes, and the structure of the reaction center has delineated the structural principles for such proteins.[5]

While UT Southwestern had played no part in supporting the body of work for which the Nobel Prize was awarded, it legitimately laid claim to having recognized Deisenhofer's considerable academic talents and recruiting him to its faculty, the pleasant Dallas winters and Kirsten Fischer-Lindahl notwithstanding!

✳ ✳ ✳ ✳ ✳

During his first year as dean, Wildenthal appointed committees to recommend priorities for the next decade of development in education, research, and clinical practice. "After meeting for about six months, all of these committees identified building a University Hospital for private patients as the most urgent priority for the school," he stated. "But I knew that the Board of Regents of the UT System was not likely to dedicate state funds for such a purpose and that we would have to go to the private sector to raise money for a private hospital."[1] As a result, a dialogue was cultivated between the leadership at UT Southwestern and the Dallas community, a dialogue that spawned not only the establishment of the Zale Lipshy University Hospital in 1989, but led to an enhanced level of community involvement with the medical center that, over the next decade, generated over $1 billion in philanthropic contributions for research, education, and clinical programs. Given that the state had fallen on hard times in 1986, the timing could not have been more propitious.

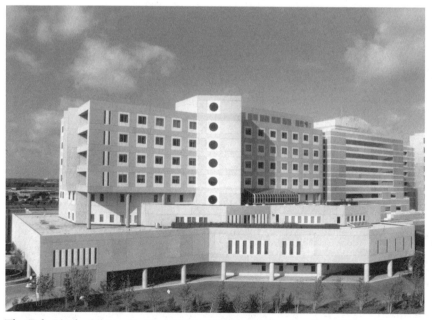

The Zale Lipshy University Hospital opened in 1990 as the first UT Southwestern University Hospital.

CHAPTER 9

PORTRAITS OF SOME PROMINENT DALLAS PHILANTHROPISTS

The roots of the decision to build a university hospital in the early 1980s can be traced to events in the 1970s that included the near collapse of the Department of Surgery at Southwestern, and, not coincidentally, of Parkland Hospital. Wildenthal explains how this situation developed.

> In the early 1970s several of the clinical departments were strong at Parkland. But we were small and relatively weak in many surgical sub-specialties, such as ophthalmology, orthopedics, neurosurgery and otolaryngology—activities that required a significant number of referral patients to achieve a critical mass. However, there was no hospital to refer such patients to in adequate numbers. Parkland was (and still is) a hospital primarily dedicated to serving the indigent community of Dallas County and dealing with medical emergencies and was not suitable for building a referral practice for elective patients. This was the principal issue that led Tom Shires to resign the chair of surgery and depart to Washington University in 1974, taking about two-thirds of the surgeons with him and leaving Parkland barely manned, let alone strong. Shires had campaigned aggressively for a private outpatient clinic and a private hospital at the medical school. But there were no obvious sources of funds to achieve these goals. The state was still giving us healthy increases, but not for those purposes. And a private hospital was simply not a realistic school priority then.[1]

This aggravating situation was compounded by Parkland's continuing physical deterioration; the hospital was in a crisis mode by the end of the 1970s. "Parkland was starved for funds, it was run down and it was poorly managed," Wildenthal related. "It literally ran out of money in its bank account every July or August and would have to survive on a line of credit from the banks. It was impossible to build under such circumstances."[1] Relief came when Dallas

County voters approved an $80 million bond orchestrated by Ralph Rogers for a new physical facility (see chapter 7).

These experiences served as an urgent wake-up call; by the early 1980s, a consensus had been reached that the university should acquire its own private hospital to which patients in the surgical subspecialties could be referred. "In those days the Board of Regents of the University of Texas was in no mood to allow a state facility to own and operate another hospital, particularly in light of negative financial experiences with such ventures in Galveston and Tyler," Wildenthal explained. "So we knew we would have to turn to the private sector."

In 1982, Sprague and Wildenthal began discussions with the Zale and Lipshy families. Donald Zale was largely responsible for the huge growth of the Zale Corporation, a business started as the Zale Jewelry Company in 1924 by his father Morris that is today one of the world's largest jewelry distributors. Don Zale worked for the Zale Corporation for thirty-five years, rising to the positions of chairman and CEO. When Morris Zale retired as president of the Zale Jewelry Company in 1957, his brother-in-law Ben Lipshy succeeded him.

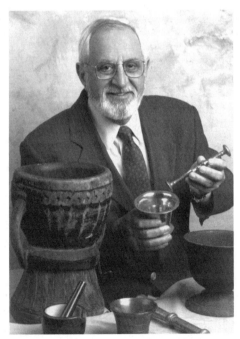

Robert (Bob) Kramer, a Dallas pediatrician, brought about a meeting between UT Southwestern and Donald Zale and Bruce Lipshy.

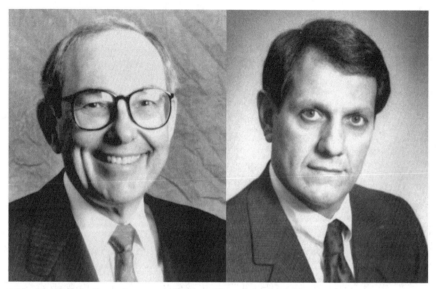

Donald Zale (left) and Bruce Lipshy (right), after whom the Zale Lipshy Hospital is named.

During the 1970s, Lipshy's son Bruce became vice-president of the Zale Corporation, and his cousin Don Zale served as president.

"Don Zale and Bruce Lipshy came to us through the mediation of their mutual friend Bob Kramer,"[1] Wildenthal commented. A private Dallas pediatrician, Kramer was an ardent supporter of academic medicine. Firm in the belief that a great medical school required a great university hospital, he had long been enthusiastic about moving the Children's Medical Center to the campus and linking it to the medical school. Furthermore, he told his friends Don Zale and Bruce Lipshy, who were exploring ways to appropriately memorialize their parents, about the school's urgent need. "So not too long after we had identified a university hospital as an urgent priority, but without knowing where the money might come from, Bob Kramer introduced us to the Zales and the Lipshys with this subject already in their minds,"[1] Wildenthal stated.

In the early 1980s, the hospital industry was still fairly lucrative. Sprague and Wildenthal, therefore, were reasonably confident that community contributions, including sizeable sums from the Zale and Lipshy families, would cover the costs of a new facility. "These were the pre-managed-care days, and unless a hospital was absolutely inundated with indigent patients, it could generate profits if it was competently managed," Wildenthal commented. "So revenue bond financing for part of the construction costs was reasonable to foresee."[1]

The decision to build a university hospital necessitated an additional commitment to a new outpatient facility. "If we had a private in-patient hospital we obviously had to have out-patient clinics," Wildenthal explained. "Fortunately we were able to use some state resources to help build the Aston Ambulatory Care Center."[1]

As Wildenthal explains, Southwestern could not have begun courting the Dallas community at a better time.

> When the recession hit and state funding was dramatically reduced it was imperative for us to secure alternative sources of financial support if we were to continue moving forward, not just for constructing the hospital, but also for launching new research and clinical programs and endowing faculty positions. But we had no organized inroads to the community or to our alumni at that time. We had no development office; we had no database; we didn't even have a mailing list of any substance. We had Charlie Sprague of course. Charlie enjoyed extraordinary respect in Dallas and had tremendous credibility with a small but influential group of people who were movers and shakers. But there was no sustained history of major philanthropy as far as the medical school was concerned.
>
> In 1986, when state funding dropped, we didn't have time to begin an organized community-wide campaign that might generate multiple gifts of $10,000 here and $20,000 there in sufficient volume to meet our needs. That would take years to build. We needed millions of dollars and we needed them quickly. Without a staff, or a history of this type of fundraising, it was clear that we needed to identify individuals who might make very substantial gifts and then convince them that the medical school was really worth supporting. So we had to do the obvious things—visit with people who clearly knew the medical school and also begin introducing the institution to new people. Those who both knew the institution and had the financial resources to make a difference included Harold Simmons, Ross Perot, Eric Jonsson, Cecil Green, the McDermott Foundation, and a few other individuals who preferred to remain anonymous. So beginning in early 1987, that's where we started.[1]

And to this end, Brown and Goldstein's 1985 Nobel Prize could not have been more perfectly timed. Wildenthal explains how Rogers, upon hearing the news, approached Ross Perot to ask for his support.

> The first thing that Rogers asked Perot to do, or that Perot volunteered to do, I'm not sure which, was to celebrate the Nobel Prize.

Perot was in fact himself offended that the City of Dallas would go to the trouble of sponsoring a parade for a championship football team, but didn't do anything notable for two Nobel Prize winners. So he underwrote a dinner that brought some 300 of Dallas's most influential citizens to the campus to honor the Nobel Prize. This joyous affair was especially important because it really got Perot focused on us. He had decided to do something for Brown and Goldstein, but in the process he gained confidence that the entire institution really was a world-class operation.[1]

Wildenthal proved to be an excellent fundraiser. In the two decades between 1986 and 2005, his efforts generated almost $2 billion in gifts and pledges, half of which are in endowment funds. It is unlikely that any other U.S. medical school has fared as well. Wildenthal's secret is deceptively simple and straightforward—he "sells" premier quality.

Dallas is a philanthropic community—and a wealthy community. But in fundraising it's important to link disposable wealth to causes of outstanding quality. Money can sometimes be raised for second-rate causes. But one can't do that sort of thing again and again. So it's important to ask people to support only first-rate programs. That is absolutely essential as far as I am concerned. Another crucial aspect of fundraising is that donors must acquire a sense of confidence that the projects they donate money for are thoughtfully monitored, that their goals are adhered to, and that the funds are entrusted to reliable people. One has to not only have good researchers, good clinicians and good teachers in an institution, but also good business management and good feedback, so that people understand that their contributions have really made a difference. That's the long term secret of successful fund raising.[1]

Steve McKnight, Joe Sambrook's successor as head of the Department of Biochemistry since 1996, enthusiastically endorsed Wildenthal's view. McKnight was born and raised in Texas, earned his PhD at the University of Virginia, and was appointed a Howard Hughes Investigator at the Carnegie Institution in Washington, DC—all the while keeping a watchful eye on UT Southwestern. When he decided to leave the Carnegie Institution in the early 1990s, he came close to joining the Southwestern faculty, but finally decided instead to help establish a private biotechnology company in California. "At that time of my life founding the company that we called Tularik was an exciting adventure that I simply didn't want to pass up."[2] Tularik, founded by McKnight and

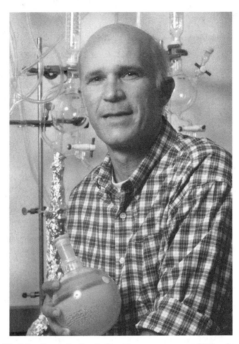

Steven (Steve) McKnight has chaired the Department of Biochemistry since 1996. McKnight was elected to the U.S. National Academy of Sciences in 1992.

his colleagues Robert Tjian and Dave Goedell, is now a thriving drug discovery and development company in San Francisco.

Not long after McKnight and his family had settled in California, William B. (Bill) Neaves, Wildenthal's successor as dean of the medical school, visited. "Bill told me with quiet determination and confidence that he fully expected me to end up at Southwestern once Tularik was on its feet. Brown and Goldstein were equally adamant. [Both had agreed to serve on the company's scientific advisory board]. This continued interest by the UT Southwestern leadership impressed me a lot."[2] By 1995, McKnight agreed to join Southwestern's full-time faculty as chairman (Sambrook had already left for Australia) while remaining part-time at Tularik.

As McKnight explains, his recruitment was significantly facilitated by a financial package provided by an anonymous philanthropic patron.

A lot of well meaning philanthropists become bamboozled by the numerous pitches that are made to them, and often their money ends up supporting second rate stuff. But this anonymous donor, and other big donors in Dallas, are very astute about making sure that their

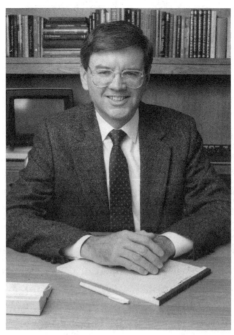

William B. Neaves, Dean of UT Southwestern Medical School from 1989–1998. Neaves also served as Dean of the School of Graduate Studies from 1980–1986.

money supports real quality. And this is the critical role that Kern plays so well. He cultivates philanthropy in a professional manner. Kern cares that philanthropic monies are well spent. If donors observe that their funds are supporting the very best programs, it's tremendously helpful in ensuring that money continues to flow. When philanthropy is used to help band-aid programs that can't otherwise get funded, or if donors get carried away with science that sounds good to them but that one knows doesn't really have a future, it eventually backfires. Kern understands this. He identifies donors, educates them, gets to know them, and generates sustained relationships with them. I'll bet there's no one in the country who can match him at this.

Consider the impact of the Endowed Scholar Program and how quality has ensured the success of the program.* This program not

---

* Now in its ninth year, the Endowed Scholar Program in Biomedical Research provides in excess of $1,000,000 over four years to five first-time, tenure-track assistant professors at The University of Texas Southwestern Medical Center at Dallas. Funded by pri-

only allows us to recruit outstanding young faculty members every year [by providing substantial start-up packages], some of whom will likely represent the next generation of scientific leadership here, but since nominations for these positions come directly out of individual departments to a central committee that selects the scholars, it has encouraged academic departments to search for the very best young faculty, knowing that only the best and brightest will qualify for support by this richly endowed program.[2]

* * * * *

I pointedly asked Wildenthal whether philanthropy was a fundamental cultural phenomenon in Texas. He replied:

There is definitely a culture of 'giving back' throughout Texas. But it's an especially strong phenomenon in Dallas, Houston and Fort Worth. Certainly in Dallas it's been engrained in the business and social establishments that if one wants to be respected in this community one needs to give back in one way or another, either by volunteering to raise money or by giving it directly. There is a definite spirit in Dallas—and this would be true for all of Texas—that we want to be recognized for being as good as anybody else, if not better. It's a sort of frontier, entrepreneurial spirit I think. The feeling is very much that if we want to play in the big leagues we have to have institutions comparable to Harvard and Yale and Stanford—and the Metropolitan Opera, and the Philadelphia Orchestra, and Art Museum of Chicago. I think that it is fair to say that over the past 20 years or so, certainly with the Nobel Prizes that have come our way, the civic leadership in Dallas has come to realize that UT Southwestern is truly recognized world-wide.[1]

McKnight concurs. "There's definitely a can-do spirit in this city. If Dallas has a football team it wants it to be the best. If it has a symphony it must be the best and housed in the best concert hall. And if we're going to have a medical school here let's make that the best, too."[2]

When Perot finally met with Goldstein and Brown to discuss how he might support the medical school, he was surprised with their suggestion. While they were indeed eager to have him support their research on cholesterol, they were more concerned that he devote his resources both to young faculty members

---

vate endowment, the program has already assured the successful launch of research careers for a cadre of 45 young and creative investigators.

and to helping the school attract the best possible graduate students. "After discussions that lasted the better part of a year with lots of conversation back and forth, Perot contributed an extraordinarily generous three-part package to the school over the long term," Wildenthal recounted. "Research support was provided directly to Brown and Goldstein. Additionally, support was provided for a small group of faculty selected by Brown and Goldstein, who would work under their direct mentorship, though not on the same problems as they were tackling. The third and largest component of Perot's contribution was to strengthen the existing MD/PhD program at the school, the Medical Scientist Training Program (MSTP)."[1]

The value of upgrading the MSTP is incalculable. The program, instituted by the NIH in 1964, was designed to foster the emergence of a group of physicians who would pursue careers in academic medicine and tackle human disease problems at a fundamental level. The nationwide program provided financial support to students while they completed both their MD and PhD training. The best medical schools could compete for annual support for a maximum of three to six applicants. Perot's contribution enabled UT Southwestern to mount the single largest program in the country, admitting as many as fifteen outstandingly qualified students from around the country. Between 1978, when the program was initiated, and 2006, the program graduated 117

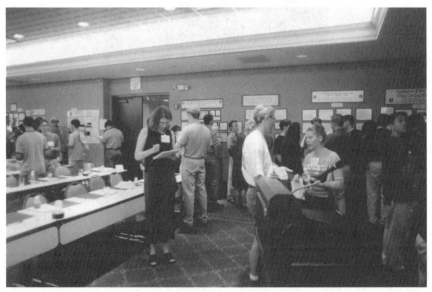

UT Southwestern students in the Medical Scientist Training Program (MSTP) enjoy the annual scientific retreat at Lake Texoma.

individuals with MD and PhD degrees, many of whom now occupy academic positions in leading biomedical research centers.

＊ ＊ ＊ ＊ ＊

Harold and Annette Simmons are two more prominent and enduring supporters of UT Southwestern. A native Texan, Harold Simmons is the son of rural schoolteachers. After graduating from UT Austin in 1952 with a master's degree in economics, Simmons borrowed money to purchase a small drugstore, using his entire $5,000 savings as a down payment. Within a decade he had built a statewide drugstore chain worth over $50 million. Simmons sold the chain in 1973 and launched a career as an investor. He now controls numerous companies, including five corporations listed on the New York Stock Exchange. In 1988 Simmons established the Harold C. Simmons Foundation, for which he serves as chairman with two of his daughters as co-trustees. His commitment of $41 million to UT Southwestern in 1988 ranked

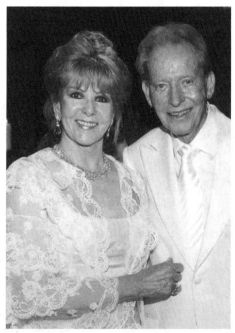

Dallas entrepreneur Harold C. Simmons and his wife Annette have provided extensive support to establish a nationally recognized cancer program at UT Southwestern.

as the largest philanthropic gift in Dallas history at the time, and was one of the largest gifts ever made for medical research in the United States.

Simmons' wife Annette, a graduate of Southern Methodist University, has served on a variety of civic organizations, including the boards of the National Kidney Foundation of Texas, the Parkland Foundation, the Susan G. Komen Breast Cancer Foundation, and the Crystal Charity Ball. Her community involvement has earned her numerous awards, including the Crystal Charity Ball Hall of Fame Award in 1997 and the Dallas County Medical Society Alliance's Champ Award in 2003. She and her husband received Southwestern Medical Foundation's Charles Cameron Sprague Community Service Award in 1995 and the Annette G. Strauss Humanitarian Award in 2000.

✳ ✳ ✳ ✳ ✳

While researching for this book, I had the pleasure of talking with a few of Southwestern's major donors. Peter O'Donnell, Jr., a prominent Dallas businessman, was born in Dallas and attended public school in Highland Park. He earned a Bachelor of Science degree from the University of the South, a small

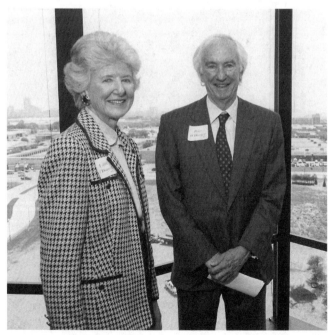

Peter and Edith O'Donnell, long-time supporters of UT Southwestern Medical Center and founders of the O'Donnell Foundation.

liberal arts college in Sewanee, Tennessee, and obtained his MBA from the Wharton Graduate School of Finance at the University of Pennsylvania before returning to Dallas to pursue his career. For over four decades, O'Donnell has sought to promote excellence in the Texas educational system. In 1985 he was appointed by Governor Mark White to the Texas Select Committee on Higher Education, a working group that generated numerous reforms in colleges and universities. In 1956, O'Donnell and his wife, Edith, established the O'Donnell Foundation, with the philanthropic goals of building excellence in science and engineering programs in Texas universities, preparing more high school graduates to earn college degrees, and making outstanding arts education programs available.

O'Donnell first encountered UT Southwestern Medical School in the mid-1950s when his high school friend Philip O'Bryan Montgomery, Jr., a faculty member in the Department of Pathology (see chapter 4), approached him for help in purchasing a piece of equipment for Dr. Carleton Chapman, then

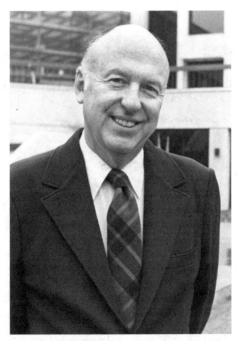

Philip O'Brien (P.O.B.) Montgomery, Jr. (1921–2005) was a long-time faculty member in the Department of Pathology at UT Southwestern. Montgomery served as a special assistant to the President's office for many years and helped orchestrate the North Campus initiative.

Chief of Cardiology in the Department of Internal Medicine. After meeting with Chapman to learn about the equipment, O'Donnell personally donated funds. Soon after, the O'Donnell Foundation provided its first formal contribution to UT Southwestern ($5,000) to support Montgomery's research program. "Phil was a great spokesman for the university," O'Donnell commented. He got an innumerable number of people interested in the medical school. "In particular he got the Texas Instruments crowd, Eric Jonsson, Eugene McDermott, and Cecil Green, involved. In my opinion this was pivotal for the school."[3] O'Donnell is reticent about discussing his own contributions (he seeks anonymity for most of his philanthropic activities), consistently deflecting credit to others such as the Texas Instrument group, Ralph Rogers, the Southwestern Medical Foundation, Ross Perot, Charlie Seay, and Harold Simmons. But he has no hesitation about discussing accountability. "A lot of our decisions are based on faith, of course—faith in individuals and faith in programs that we back at the medical school. But above and beyond that we document everything in writing. This clarifies our own thinking about what we're trying to accomplish, and sometimes it also clarifies the thinking of our recipients. And we ask for and receive formal annual reports. Of course we haven't always backed winners. We've provided support to programs that haven't performed as we thought they might. But we don't keep doing that!"[3]

O'Donnell believes that educational institutions should receive support from their communities and alumni—and not just in times of urgent need.

The University of Texas in Austin (another major beneficiary of the O'Donnell Foundation) only obtained its first endowed chair in the late 1950s. That's ridiculous. The university must have over 400,000 alumni and many of them are worth a lot of money. But for a long time they were never asked for help. I think that the general feeling was that the legislature would continue to provide. But of course that isn't always the case. Besides, there can never be enough money for important causes. We know that even when our foundation gives a lot to a program, it's really miniscule relative to the needs of that program. So we look on ourselves as providing the margin of excellence, and as assistants in recruiting the best people. Yes, we provide funds for equipment and that sort of thing. But it's really people that we invest in—because it's people that make the difference. Kern Wildenthal and Charlie Sprague told us that they needed to build molecular biology at the medical school and that they had identified Joe Sambrook to spearhead this effort. Well, Joe turned out to be a fabulous recruiter. He's a good example of why basically we bet on the jockies. It doesn't

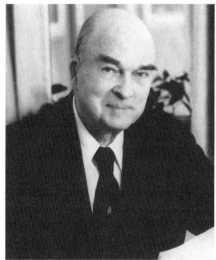
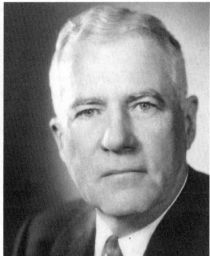
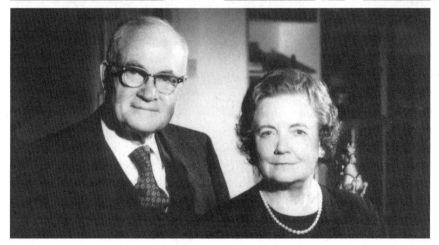

Prominent Dallas philanthropists and civic leaders. John Eric Jonsson (1901–1955) (top left) one of the co-founders of Texas Instruments (TI), Eugene McDermott (1899–1973) (top right) another co-founder of TI, and Cecil Green (1899–2003) and Ida Green (bottom). Cecil Green was the third co-founder of TI.

make much difference how they ride the horse. As long as they know how to ride well![3]

O'Donnell talked about UT Southwestern presidents and their fundraising styles.

I was on a committee to select the next president of UT Southwestern after Charlie Sprague stepped down. When we considered Kern, the question was raised about how effective he would be in raising money for the school. I have to say now that in retrospect we seriously underestimated him. The fact is that people trust Kern, and that's fundamental to fundraising. Kern engenders trust and confidence—and that's why people write the big checks.[3]

O'Donnell reluctantly discussed two of the many contributions his foundation made to the medical school. One was the Endowed Scholar Program mentioned above. "This program is very competitive, and it provides a powerful mechanism for bringing in new potential leadership in the basic sciences."[3] According to McKnight, the program has made an incalculable difference to the strength of the basic science ranks at the junior faculty level. Traditionally, individual departments are required to identify financial resources for recruiting outstanding young scientists, often a daunting challenge when stellar recruits are receiving multiple offers. Since 1999, the endowment established by the O'Donnell Foundation (and several other donors) has provided five start-up packages annually, each worth as much as a million dollars. UT Southwestern, therefore, has huge leverage when recruiting rising stars. O'Donnell also explained how the foundation helped establish electronic medical records at the hospitals and outpatient facilities. "This is going to be a long-term deal, and we're just at the beginning. But it's fundamental to the future."[3]

O'Donnell adamantly supports the notion that giving back is part of the Texan tradition. "There are a lot of successful people in this state who started out with literally nothing. Many of these folks are now motivated to give back. And they are additionally motivated to give to the medical school. Because what happens in a medical school has the potential for impacting the lives of a lot of people—especially in a great medical school such as this one."[3]

✳ ✳ ✳ ✳ ✳

Most Americans well know the name H. Ross Perot, the computer giant, philanthropist and independent candidate for the Presidency of the United States in 1992 and 1996. A native Texan, Perot was born on June 27, 1930, and attended Texas public schools and Texarkana Junior College. From early childhood on, he exercised his keen entrepreneurial skills. A biographical source indicates that "at age seven Perot started working at various jobs … including breaking horses, selling Christmas cards, magazines, and garden seeds, buying and selling bridles, saddles, horses and calves, delivering newspapers, and collecting for classified ads."[4] In 1953 he graduated from the U.S. Naval Academy and served at sea for four years on a destroyer and an aircraft carrier. In 1956 Perot married Margot Birmingham, from Greensburg, Pennsylvannia,

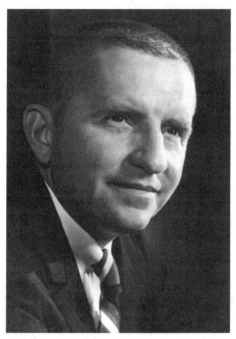

Henry Ross Perot, Dallas civic leader, computer businessman and philanthropist.

whom he met while at the Naval Academy. The couple settled in Dallas, where Ross Perot worked for IBM's data processing division as a salesman.

In 1962, Margot loaned her husband $1,000 to start Electronic Data Systems (EDS), a one-man data processing company that Perot turned into a multi-billion dollar corporation. When two EDS employees were taken hostage by the Iranian government in the late 1970s, Perot orchestrated a rescue mission led by retired Green Beret Colonel Arthur "Bull" Simons, an escapade that was dramatized by Ken Follett in his best-selling novel *On Wings of Eagles.*[4*]

I met with Perot in his sumptuous office at the new EDS headquarters in Plano, Texas, an office filled with all manner of treasures accumulated over the years. An avid collector of paintings, books, and manuscripts, Perot bought a copy of the Magna Carta in 1984, "the only copy allowed to be taken out of Great Britain. Perot loaned the document to the National Archives in

---

* When once asked by the *Dallas Morning News* how he would write his own epitaph, Perot replied: "Made more money faster. Lost more money in one day. Led the biggest jailbreak in history. He died."[4]

Washington, DC, for display alongside the U.S. Constitution and the Bill of Rights."[4]

A man with a piercing, intelligent gaze and a direct, no-nonsense demeanor, Perot related how he became involved with UT Southwestern Medical School when Brown and Goldstein received the Nobel Prize in 1985. Echoing Wildenthal's sentiments, Perot was offended that Dallas was doing nothing to honor their achievement.

> So I talked with the medical school and suggested that we have a dinner for them. Not too long after that dinner I had a chance encounter with Mike and Joe in Dallas. I asked then what they were up to and they replied that they were trying to raise funds for their research. My exact words to them were, 'Nobel Prize winners shouldn't have to wander around raising funds.' They laughed and replied that they indeed did have to raise funds, Nobel laureates or not. So I told them that they should call me any time that they needed funds—as long as they were still doing great work. They again laughed and told me that that was not the way research usually got funded! But I replied that that's the way I do things. And to this day I'm still sending them checks![5]

As already mentioned, in addition to supporting Brown and Goldstein's research program (and those of several other faculty members), Perot helped establish what is possibly the largest MSTP in the country, a program that brings about fifteen outstanding MD/PhD students to Dallas each year. Not only does Perot provide financial support to help with recruiting, but he personally attends dinners for potential MSTP students to lend his own considerable powers of persuasion.

* * * * *

Mary McDermott Cook is the daughter of Margaret and the late Eugene McDermott, another prominent Dallas philanthropist. A native of New York, Eugene obtained one master's degree in engineering from a leading technological university, the Stevens Institute of Technology in Hoboken, New Jersey, and a second master's degree from Columbia University. In 1925, he joined Everette Lee DeGolyer's Geophysical Research Corporation in Houston as a field supervisor. In 1930, DeGolyer financed McDermott and John C. Karcher in their organization of Geophysical Services Incorporated (GSI). The company soon became one of the world's foremost geophysical service firms. McDermott moved to Dallas to serve as vice-president of GSI, eventually becoming president and then chairman. In 1941, he joined with Eric Jonsson and Cecil Green to establish Texas Instruments (TI). GSI ultimately became a wholly

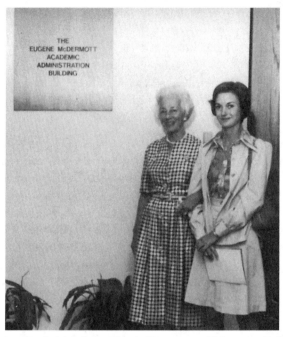

Mary McDermott Cook (right) daughter of Eugene and Margaret (left) McDermott, and president of the Eugene McDermott Foundation.

owned subsidiary of the new firm. McDermott served as TI's chairman until 1958, and remained a director until his death in 1973.

Like O'Donnell, McDermott became involved with the medical school because of his association with Philip Montgomery. And McDermott, too, believed in backing good people. Mary McDermott Cook recounted her father's introduction to the medical school.

> Dad was approached by Philip for help to purchase a research instrument that cost about $5,000," Mary McDermott related. "Dad turned him down. Not too much later Philip approached him again, this time to help bring a British scientist to work in Dallas. The cost of this was more than $5,000, but my father (Mr. Mac as he was often referred to) readily agreed. When asked why he was willing to spend more money when he had previously turned down the request for $5,000, Dad replied that he believed in people. My father always invested in brains.[6]

With his engineering background, McDermott was generally interested in "how things are put together and how they work."[6] He became particularly interested in somatotyping, a discipline devoted to the study of different body forms, and keenly followed the work of somatotyping pioneer William Sheldon.

After his wife underwent surgery at UT Southwestern in the late 1950s, Mc-Dermott established an endowed chair in anesthesiology, only the second such endowment at the medical school. His interest in the school continued—he admired Sprague and supported his programs.

> Charlie was a builder and Dad believed in building—and he thought that Charlie was the right man at the right time. Dad was the ultimate giver. He would sometimes complain that there were so many good causes to give to; his main concern was that he would run out of time before he ran out of money. But he only gave to quality."[6] Shortly before he died, McDermott's foundation, the Biological Humanics Foundation (established in the mid-1950s), founded the Eugene McDermott Center for the Study of Human Growth and Development at UT Southwestern.[6]

Eugene McDermott's capable daughter Mary and wife Margaret have continued his advocacy and support of UT Southwestern. As detailed in the next chapter, Mary McDermott Cook played a key role in the acquisition of the land on which the extensive North Campus now resides.

The importance of philanthropic and other private contributions to UT Southwestern's growth and success cannot be overstated. Numerous visitors from other leading academic medical centers have expressed their admiration—and sometimes their frank envy—at the role that the Southwestern Medical Foundation has played in the history of the medical school in Dallas. I know of no other academic institution that enjoys the level of nurturing and support that UT Southwestern enjoys from the foundation, not only in terms of direct financial contributions, but perhaps more importantly, in terms of its close ties with and continued interest in the school.

CHAPTER 10

THE NORTH CAMPUS DEVELOPMENT: A SHOWPIECE FOR THE FUTURE

For many years, a tract of land just north of the medical school lay dormant. This open space, occupying close to sixty-five acres in an otherwise highly populated urban development, initially belonged to the John D. and Catherine T. MacArthur Foundation, "a private, independent grant-making institution dedicated to helping groups and individuals foster lasting improvement in the human condition."[1] Initially, UT Southwestern had no particular interest in the space. But as the school (including the Medical Center that incorporated the medical school, its associated graduate school, and the School of Allied Health Sciences) grew, it found itself land-locked. It was unable to acquire land directly across the street from the main campus on Harry Hines Boulevard, and a federal edict precluded building on eight acres on the main campus that has been home to a population of snowy egrets since the 1950s, when they were displaced by the re-channeling of the nearby Trinity River.

In 1986, Kern Wildenthal had lunch with Mary McDermott-Cook and other members of the Biological Humanics Foundation.

> Bill Neaves and I were at the board meeting to report on the gifts the foundation had provided to date and on general progress at the school. At one point Margaret McDermott and her daughter Mary asked us what we thought was the biggest challenge facing the institution as we looked to the future. My immediate answer was that we were land-locked. I told them that while this was not a very pressing need in the late 1980s, it clearly would become so if we didn't begin thinking about this issue soon. They asked the obvious question 'Where could you possibly expand to?' I replied that the only open space in the area was the land at Harry Hines and Inwood in front of Exchange Park. I told them that we had not yet explored the

availability of the land, which we understood was owned by the MacArthur Foundation in Chicago. Providentially, one of the board members at the luncheon, Mickey LeMaistre, a former faculty member at UT Southwestern who served as Chancellor for Health Affairs in the UT System and subsequently as President of The University of Texas MD Anderson Cancer Center, informed us that he was a good friend of the President of the MacArthur Foundation, a man who used to be Chancellor of the University of Illinois System when he (LeMaistre) was Chancellor in the University of Texas System. LeMaistre enthusiastically agreed that acquisition of that land by UT Southwestern would clearly put it to very good use and offered to introduce us to the MacArthur Foundation.[2]

Vin Prothro, a civic leader who was helping the medical school develop biotechnology, volunteered to facilitate negotiations with the MacArthur Foundation. Before long, Wildenthal, Neaves, Prothro, and Philip Montgomery III (P.O.B. Montgomery, Jr.'s son) visited the foundation to explore acquiring the land as a philanthropic gift. Wildenthal explains their initial failure and subsequent success.

The president of the foundation warmed to the idea immediately and pledged to do his best. But he warned us that the MacArthur Foundation had established a ten-year strategic plan and that except for a commitment to treating and preventing parasitic diseases in the Third World, medical research was not part of that plan. He suggested that we nonetheless submit a formal proposal. We did so and a few months later received the disappointing news that the foundation's board had decided that as worthy as our proposed project was, and even though they agreed that this was indeed very good use of that land from a philanthropic point of view, it was so out of the pattern of what they wished to support that they had no choice but to turn us down.

Disappointed as we were, when we reevaluated the situation we decided to approach this issue as a business proposition with the Foundation rather than as a pure philanthropic contribution. But our options were limited. For one thing, the school was seriously strapped for cash and we couldn't afford to buy it outright. So we went to their real estate asset management division and proposed that they donate part of the land to us and allow us to purchase some of the remainder over a period of time at a discounted rate. In return we pledged to conduct all future development in our research enterprise on that land, which would both upgrade the neighborhood and considerably increase the value of the land that they retained. After extended negotiations the MacArthur Foundation agreed to this transaction. The value of the land they retained was calculated to increase in value to the extent that on their books the entire transaction was a wash. On our books the transaction was partially a gift and partially a bargain purchase that was stretched over a period of years.[2]

With the Inwood Road site secured, a long-term building plan was developed and Wildenthal set about securing funding. Once again, Dallas philanthropists stepped forward. "At about that time Harold Simmons was contemplating a substantial gift to UT Southwestern," Wildenthal explained. "He ultimately made a $41 million commitment, which included funds towards the first North Campus building, now called the Simmons Building. Subsequently Nancy Hamon and Charles and Sarah Seay made substantial gifts that facilitated the erection of two more buildings appropriately named for them."[2]

In 2003 the Moncrief Radiation Oncology Building was donated by W. A. "Tex" Moncrief and in 2005, a fifth building, an imposing fourteen-story fa-

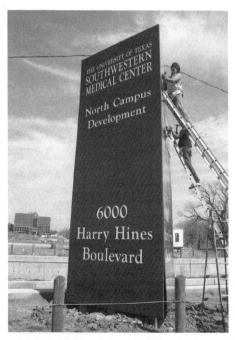

The UT Southwestern Medical Center North Campus began development in the early 1990s.

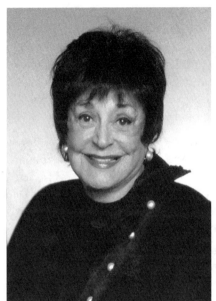 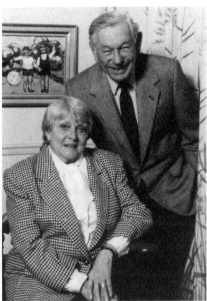

Nancy Hamon (left), a prominent Dallas philanthropist for whom the Hamon Building on the North Campus is named, and Charles and Sarah Seay (right) Dallas civic leaders and philanthropists for whom the Seay Building on the North Campus is named.

cility that rises majestically over the campus, opened its doors. A year later the Bill and Rita Clements Advanced Medical Imaging Building, named for former Texas Governor William P. "Bill" Clements, Jr. and his wife Rita (a member of the Board of Regents of the University of Texas System), completed the so-called phase one ensemble. All six buildings are interconnected, once again assuring vertical and horizontal contiguity between 1.5 million square feet of academic space.

With the opening of the first buildings on the North Campus, the medical center physically embraced a facility dating back to 1898 when the Sisters of St. Vincent de Paul opened the St. Paul Hospital—a six-story building distinguished as the first fireproof structure in Dallas. Operated as a private facility for many years, St. Paul Hospital was purchased by UT Southwestern Medical Center in 2000 and leased to Zale Lipshy University Hospital so that it could be operated as a second patient referral site. In 2005 the trustees deeded the two hospitals to UT Southwestern and they became formally integrated components of UT Southwestern Medical Center.

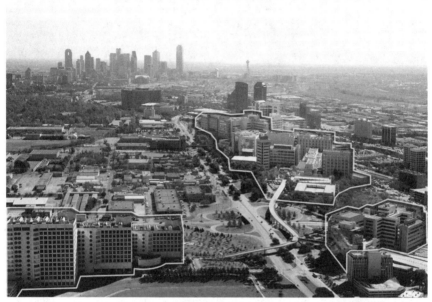

An aerial view of the UT Southwestern campus circa 2006. The buildings shown at the bottom left are the new north campus. The private road for the transportation shuttle can be seen snaking its way from the North Campus over Harry Hines Blvd to the St. Paul UT Southwestern University Hospital complex (bottom right) and then to the south campus. Downtown Dallas is in the distance.

The growth of UT Southwestern Medical Center at Dallas has by no means been limited to academic and clinical buildings. Cognizant of the need to house graduate students and postdoctoral research fellows close to the laboratories in which they spend their waking (and many of their sleeping) hours, the university acquired a vacant parcel of land just north of the campus and erected apartment blocks—the Southwestern Medical Park Apartments. Student life was further enriched with the construction of the Bryan Williams, MD Student Center on the South Campus, a 43,000 square foot facility outfitted for physical activities including basketball, badminton and volleyball, as well as special events such as student functions and parents' day. As this book went to press, plans were rapidly evolving for the next generation of research facilities and for consolidation and expansion of the entire clinical enterprise. The anticipated physical dimensions of the medical center during the next several decades are nothing short of astounding, projecting the erection of 2.5 million nsf of additional research space on the North Campus, and the construction

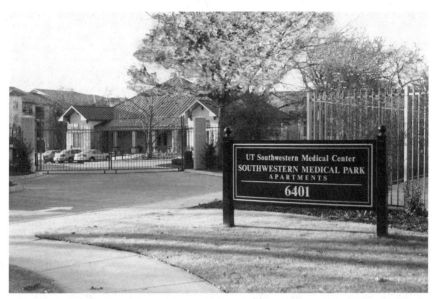

The UT Southwestern Medical Park Apartments on Mockingbird Road. These provide convenient access to the medical center for students, fellows, interns and residents.

of multiple clinical towers where the St. Paul UT Southwestern University Hospital is presently located. The first of these clinical towers is already rising.

The transformation from countryside housing army barracks to multiple acres of glass and concrete structures over a period of little more than half a century is surely nothing short of a phenomenal rise from rags to riches.

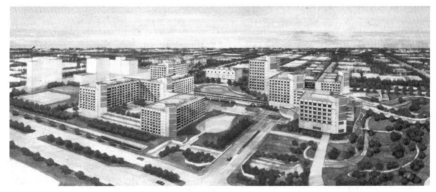

An artist's rendition of the future North Campus showing the existing research complex on the right and the proposed second phase of research buildings on the left.

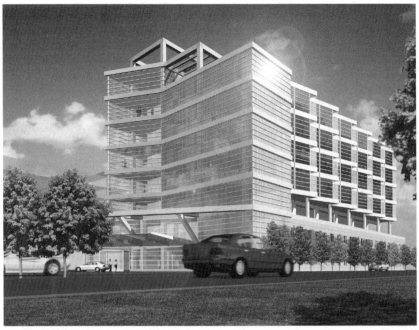

An artist's rendition of the proposed future complex of medical towers at the site of the present St. Paul University Hospital.

CHAPTER 11

EPILOGUE

There is no question that UT Southwestern Medical Center has secured a position of leadership in American medicine. It now boasts a 230-acre facility with affiliates in Dallas, Frisco, Richardson, Fort Worth, Waco, and Wichita Falls, and an annual operating budget of well over a billion dollars. The institution renders health care to over 90,000 inpatients and 2 million outpatients every year. The three degree-granting schools—the School of Medicine, the Graduate School of Biomedical Sciences, and the School of Allied Health Sciences—collectively train over 4,000 students, residents, and postdoctoral fellows annually, including over 100 students in the Medical Scientist Training (combined MD/PhD) Program. At the time of this writing annual support for biomedical research from federal and other granting agencies stands at an impressive $300 million.

Despite such success, however, the Medical Center cannot rest on its laurels. The complexion of both biomedical research and academic medical practice are rapidly changing, and the institution, like others around the country, confronts formidable challenges as it moves forward in the 21st century.

In the research arena, the academic community is facing unprecedented opportunities—and alarming risks. The golden age of molecular biology that began in the middle of the 20th century and quickly gained staggering momentum laid enduring foundations for applying our knowledge of basic biology to the understanding and treatment of human disease. Effective translation of research from the laboratory to the bedside, however, demands expensive and logistically challenging interdisciplinary and multi-disciplinary efforts. Continued support of these endeavors will require massive resources not readily available at all U.S. academic institutions. Choices will have to be made, weighing risks of success against costs. Will stem cell research truly deliver on the phenomenal promises of regenerative medicine? Will gene expression profiling and clinical proteomics revolutionize the diagnosis and treatment of cancer? Will gene therapy become a routine reality for eliminating the scourge of devastating hereditary diseases? Incorrectly guessing the answers to these and many other questions that now grace the editorial pages of the biomedical literature may turn out to be prohibitively costly—at many levels.

Large multi-disciplinary research projects bring other complexities to the ivory tower. Donald Kennedy, editor-in-chief of the influential weekly journal *Science*, pointed out that whereas the number of authors per article in an issue of the journal published just five years ago averaged four, that number rose to twelve in the 2005 125th anniversary issue, with a range of two to fifty.[1] How will academic institutions accurately and fairly determine and reward individual authors on papers with fifty co-authors?

The challenges facing the *practice* of academic medicine are even more daunting. Health care costs continue to reach frightening proportions. In recent years, the U.S. has spent over $6,000 per person annually, a sum that translates to a staggering sixteen percent of the gross national product. The overall cost of health care therefore, is considerably more expensive. Yet patients not only expect (and deserve) outstanding clinical health care in the extensive network of private facilities, they also expect academic medical centers to deliver the same overall quality of service. Meeting such service expectations and demands presents formidable challenges to the culture of academic medicine, a culture in which practicing clinicians are philosophically wedded to teaching and training medical students and residents, traveling to medical and scientific conferences, and conducting research. Moreover, given the imperative for increasing attention to the financial bottom line, clinical departments in academic medical centers may give thought to embracing physicians with business skills that are as well honed as their clinical skills, and medical schools may have to find ways to incorporate such training in their already impossibly jammed curricula.

Such commercialization is fraught with risks that threaten to undermine the very fabric of academia, and debate rages on the wisdom of embracing these strategic shifts. While on the one hand "proponents applaud universities and colleges becoming more relevant in strengthening America's competitive position in a global innovation economy—and more efficient or accountable in the process, [on the other hand] [o]pponents point to increasing conflicts of interest, profit-driven decision-making, and corporate influence in curricula content and design as weakening academia's ability to encourage critical thinking, new ideas, spontaneous innovation and free scientific discovery."[2] In a recent book entitled *Universities in the Marketplace: The Commercialization of Higher Education,*[2] former Harvard President Derek Bok warns, "there are limits to how far a business approach can extend within the university structure. Given states' declining shares of support for higher education, the need to identify alternate funding sources may cause some schools to consider business alliances that could compromise their missions."[3]

Some academic medical centers have confronted these awesome challenges by expanding their sphere of operations in order to become or remain competitive in the clinical practice arena. Aside from the formidable costs of continued expansion, institutions that elect to follow this route will necessarily become administratively more complex. Is this a viable philosophy for UT Southwestern? Without a doubt, an increase in size and complexity would impact the unique gestalt that has long characterized the school. We must never forget that the transformation from the Oak Lawn Avenue shacks to the imposing North Campus towers was guided by a remarkable group who believed in and practiced collegiality and team spirit—men and women who shared a vision of being the best, but not necessarily the biggest. But we must also remind ourselves that the challenges for the 21st century may no longer be amenable to solution by individual entrepreneurship.

The many ethical questions now confronting the practice of medicine are equally intimidating. In time, we will all likely have our complete genetic profile available on some sort of personal identification card. Japan is already moving in this direction. Will health insurance providers, who may elect to decline insurance based on established genetic risk, have access to such information? Should women routinely have known breast cancer genes sequenced to determine their genetic risk? And if a woman is found to carry such a mutation, who should be privy to this knowledge, and what treatment should be recommended? Should such women have their breasts removed prophylactically, even though the cancer has not yet appeared? And, because women with a hereditary predisposition to breast cancer also face an increased risk of ovarian cancer, should they also have their ovaries removed as a precautionary measure? The medical profession has been confronted with difficult ethical questions such as these for some years—but definitive answers remain elusive.

The 21st century offers no shortage of challenges to the UT Southwestern Medical Center at Dallas. In principle, however, these are no more intimidating than those faced a century ago by Charles Rosser and Edward Cary when they pondered the future of academic medicine in Dallas late into the night.

Distinguished
UT Southwestern
Faculty Members

Nobel laureates

1985   Michael S. Brown, MD
1985   Joseph L. Goldstein, MD
1988   Johann Deisenhofer, PhD
1994   Alfred G. Gilman, MD, PhD

Members of the U.S. National Academy of Sciences

1979   Ronald Estabrook, PhD
1980   Michael S. Brown, MD
1980   Joseph L. Goldstein, MD
1983   Jean D. Wilson, MD
1984   Jonathan W. Uhr, MD
1985   Alfred G. Gilman, MD, PhD
1986   Roger H. Unger, MD
1992   Steven L. McKnight, PhD
1993   David Garbers, PhD
1994   Ellen S. Vitetta, PhD
1997   Johann Deisenhofer, PhD
2000   Eric N. Olson, PhD
2002   Thomas C. Südhof, MD
2003   Masashi Yanagisawa, MD, PhD
2004   Xiaodong Wang, PhD
2006   Melanie Cobb, PhD
2006   David W. Russell, PhD

Members of the Institute of Medicine of the U.S. National Academy of Sciences

1974	Donald W. Seldin, MD
1975	Ronald Estabrook, PhD
1987	Michael S. Brown, MD
1987	Joseph L. Goldstein, MD
1989	Daniel W. Foster, MD
1989	Alfred G. Gilman, MD, PhD
1994	Jean D. Wilson, MD
1995	Scott M. Grundy, MD, PhD
1997	Ron J. Anderson, MD
1998	Eric J. Nestler, MD, PhD
1998	Carol A. Tamminga, MD
1999	Kern Wildenthal, MD, PhD
2001	Norman F. Gant, MD
2001	Eric N. Olson, PhD
2004	Helen Hobbs, MD
2004	John D. McConnell, MD
2005	Steven L. McKnight, PhD
2006	George Lister. MD
2006	Ellen Vitetta, PhD

Members of the American Academy of Arts and Sciences

1974	Donald W. Seldin, MD
1981	Michael S. Brown, MD
1981	Joseph L. Goldstein, MD
1982	Jean D. Wilson, MD
1988	Alfred G. Gilman, MD, PhD
1992	Daniel W. Foster, MD
1992	David Garbers, PhD
1992	Steven L. McKnight, PhD
1993	Jonathan W. Uhr, MD
1994	Roger H. Unger, MD
1998	Eric N. Olson, PhD
2003	Ellen S. Vitetta, PhD
2005	Eric J. Nestler, MD, PhD
2006	Helen H. Hobbs, MD

NOTES

Chapter 1

1. Interview with Al Gilman.
2. http://nobelprize.org/medicine/laureates/1994/press.html.
3. *Zuckerman, H. A., Scientific Elite: Nobel Laureates in the United States.* New York: Free Press, 1977.
4. Kling, J. *UT Southwestern: From Army Shacks to Research Elites.* Science, 274: 1459-1461, 1996.

Chapter 2

1. Ludmerer, K. *Learning to Heal: The Development of American Medical Education from the Turn of the Century to the Era of Managed Care.* Oxford University Press, 2005.
2. http://www.viable-herbal.com/herbology/herbs34.htm.
3. http://www.bartleby.com/65/el/Eliot-Ch.html.
4. Flexner, A. *Medical Education in the United States and Canada.* Carnegie Foundation for the Advancement of Teaching, New York, 1910.

Chapter 3

1. Interview with Donald Seldin.
2. Mooney, B. *More Than Armies: The Story of Edward H. Cary, MD.* Mathis, Van Nort & Co. Dallas, TX, 1948.
3. *A Sense of Mission.* Parkland Memorial Hospital, 1994, special publication.
4. Fordtran, J. *Medicine in Dallas 100 years ago.* BUMC Proc 13: 34-44, 2000.
5. *Dallas Morning News.* August 15, 1900.

6. Chapman, J. S. *The University of Texas Southwestern Medical School: Medical Education in Dallas 1900-1975.* SMU Press, Dallas, TX, 1976.

7. "Letters from a Dallas medical student 1904-1907." *Legacies, A History Journal for Dallas and North Central Texas.* Spring, 1993.

8. Jackson, R. W. and F. E. Pollo. *The Legacy of Professor Adolf Lorenz.* Baylor University Medical Center Proc. 17: 3-7, 2004.

9. Flexner, A. *Medical Education in the United States and Canada.* Carnegie Foundation for the Advancement of Teaching, New York, 1910.

10. Southwestern Medical Foundation, charter.

11. Strauss, M. M., Brochure for Southwestern Medical Foundation.

12. Vanderpool, G. C. "Educating Doctors in Dallas: Dr. Edward H. Cary and the Southwestern Medical Foundation." *Legacies: A History Journal for Dallas and North Central Texas.* Spring, 1993.

13. Moursund, W. H. *A History of Baylor University College of Medicine 1900-1953.* Houston: Gulf Printing, 1956.

14. http://www.dallasnews.com/s/dws/spe/2002/hiddenhistory/1876-1900/070002dnhhparkland.448c2c57.html

Chapter 4

1. Chapman, J. S. *The University of Texas Southwestern Medical School: Medical Education in Dallas 1900-1975.* SMU Press, Dallas, TX, 1976.

2. Interview with Jean Wilson.

3. Personal communication with James Pittman, University of Alabama.

4. Montgomery Jr., P. O. B., videotape, University of Texas Southwestern Medical Center Archives.

Chapter 5

1. *Donald Wayne Seldin, MD: A conversation with the editor.* BUMC Proc. 16: 193-220, 2003.

2. http://info.med.yale.edu/intmed/history/history_page_4.html.

3. Interview with Donald Seldin.

4. Chapman, J. S. *The University of Texas Southwestern Medical School: Medical Education in Dallas 1900-1975.* SMU Press, Dallas, 1976.

5. Seldin, D. W. *Some reflections on the role of basic research and service in clinical departments.* J. Clin. Invest. 45: 976-79, 1966.

6. Personal communication with James Pittman, University of Alabama.

7. Goldstein, J. L. *Acceptance of Kobler Medal.* J. Clin. Invest, 110: S5-13, 2002.

8. Interview with Jean Wilson.

9. Wilson, J. D., *A Double Life: Academic Physician and Androgen Physiologist*, Ann. Rev. Physiol. 65: 1-21, 2003.

10. Interview with Burton Combes.

11. Interview with Michael Brown.

Chapter 6

1. http://depts.washington.edu/mednews/vol3/c1999/aagaardbio.html.

2. Chapman, J. S. *The University of Texas Southwestern Medical School: Medical Education in Dallas 1900-1975.* SMU Press, Dallas, TX, 1976.

3. Interview with Donald Seldin.

4. *Dallas Morning News.* Sept 18, 2005.

5. Charles Sprague, from *An Institution Comes of Age*, Pamela Lyon, Biologue.

6. Interview with Jean Wilson.

7. Licinio, J., P. W. Gold, G. P. Chrousos, and E. M. Sternberg, *Forty years of neuroendocrinology: a tribute to SM McCann.* Mol. Psych. 2: 347-49, 1997.

8. Interview with Ronald Estabrook.

9. Interview with Steve McKnight.

10. Interview with Jonathan Uhr.

11. Interview with Al Gilman.

12. http://nobelprize.org/medicine/laureates/1994/gilman-autobio.html.

13. Gilman, A. G. *G Proteins and Regulation of Adenylyl Cyclase.* Nobel Lectures, Physiology or Medicine 1991-1995, (ed) N. Ringertz, World Scientific Pub. Co., Singapore, 1997.

14. http://nobelprize.org/medicine/laureates/1994/rodbell

15. http://nobelprize.org/medicine/laureates/1994/presentation-speech.html.

Chapter 7

1. Rogers, R. B. *Splendid Torch.* Phoenix Publishing, West Kennebunk, ME, 1993.

2. http://nobelprize.org/medicine/laureates/1985/brown-speech.html
http://nobelprize.org/medicine/laureates/1985/goldstein-speech.html.

3. Interview with Michael Brown.

4. Brown, M. and W. G. Groves, *Intestinal Propulsion in Restrained and Unrestrained Rats*. Proc. Soc. Exp. Biol. Med. 121: 989-92, 1966.

5. Interview with Joseph Goldstein.

6. Goldstein, J. L. *Acceptance of Kobler Medal*. J. Clin. Invest, 110: S5-13, 2002.

7. http://www.nobel.se/medicine/laureates/1985/press.html.

8. Newmark, P. *Cell cholesterol wins the day*. Nature 317: 569. 1985.

9. Weissman, G. *Slighted Dallas*. Nature 318: 308, 1985.

Chapter 8

1. Interview with Kern Wildenthal.

2. Interview with Joseph Goldstein.

3. http://www.hhmi.org/about/index.html.

4. Interview with Johann Deisenhofer.

5. http://nobelprize.org/chemistry/laureates/1988/presentation-speech.html.

Chapter 9

1. Interview with Kern Wildenthal.

2. Interview with Steven McKnight.

3. Interview with Peter O'Donnell.

4. http://www.famoustexans.com/rossperot.htm

5. Interview with Ross Perot.

6. Interview with Mary McDermott.

Chapter 10

1. http://www.macfound.org/index.htm.

2. Interview with Kern Wildenthal.

Chapter 11

1. Kennedy, D. *Anniversary reflections*. Science 309: 1153, 2005.

2. Bok, D. *Universities in the Marketplace: The Commercialization of Higher Education*. Princeton Univ. Press, Princeton, NJ. 2003.

3. http://www.matr.net/article-7812.htm.

INDEX

Book, article and journal titles are in *italic* font; illustrations are indicated with **bold** font.

A

Aagaard, George, xiv, 56, **57**, 71
Academy, The. *See* U.S. National Academy of Sciences
Albright, Fuller, 53
Allen (William) Award, 122
Alpern, Robert J, xvii
AMA. *See* American Medical Association (AMA)
American Academy of Arts and Sciences, 87
  UT Southwestern faculty membership list, 170
American Chemical Society
  Pfizer Award for Enzyme Chemistry, 122
American Heart Association
  Basic Science Research Prize, 97
  Research Achievement Award, 122
American Medical Association (AMA), 28, 31
American Society for Clinical Investigation
  58th Annual Meeting, 59
  UT Southwestern faculty presentations at, 67
American Society of Human Genetics
  William Allan Award, 122
American Society of Pharmacology & Experimental Therapeutics
  Goodman and Gilman Award in Drug Receptor Pharmacology, 97
anatomy, department of

converted to department of cellular biology, 83
  Looney, 42
Anderson, Dick, 121
Anderson, Monroe D, 34
Anderson, Ron J., 170
anesthesiology
  chair endowed by McDermott, 155
animal research, 54, 90, 104–5, 111
apartments
  Southwestern Medical Park, 161, **162**
Arrowsmith, 64
Association of American Medical Colleges
  Distinguished Research Award in Biomedical Sciences, 97, 122
  Sprague as administrator, 78
Association of American Physicians
  Kobler Medal, 50
Aston Ambulatory Care Center, xvi, 140
Aston, James, 77

B

Baptist World Alliance, 29
  Pastor George W. Truett, 28
Baruch, Bernard, 106
Bass, Paul M., 97
Baylor University
  College of Medicine and Dentistry, xiii, **30**
  Hospital, xiii, 28
  Medical Center, 39
  Neff, President Pat Morris, **34**
  sectarian/nonsectarian affiliation conflict, 33–34

Baylor University, *continued*
    Truett, **29**
Beering (Steven C.) Award, 97
Bellevue Hospital Medical College, 20,
    22–23
Bernstein (Albion O.) Award, 122
Beth Israel Hospital, 73
Bigelow, Henry Jacob, 13–14
Billingham Rupert E., xv, **84**
    early medical training, 83–84
    recruited by Seldin, 84–85
biochemistry, department of, xv, xvii,
    xviii
    Estabrook, chair, 80, **81**, 83, 126
    McKnight, chair, 5, 141–**42**
    Sambrook, chair, 5, **130**, 131
    Tidwell, **42**
Biological Humanics Foundation, 155
Biomedical Research Tower, xvii
Biomedical Science, Charles C. Sprague
    Chair in, 98
Blake, Francis
    clinical scholar, 49
Bok, Derek, 166
Bonte, Fred, xv, 127
    dean, medical school, 87
    dean, UT Southwestern, **88**
Bowles, Lloyd, **80**
Brown, Alice, 110
Brown, E.R., 32–33
Brown, Michael S., xii, xv, xvi, **102, 103,
    108, 118**
    American Academy of Arts and Sci-
        ences member, 170
    awards shared with Goldstein, 122
    collaboration with Goldstein, 101,
        115–17, 119–20
    HMG-CoA reductase, 111–12, 114
    Institute of Medicine member, 170
    internship and residency with Gold-
        stein, 108–9
    Journal of Biological Chemistry, 114
    medical education, 104–5
    mentored by Siperstein, 65
    NIH research commission, 109–11
    Nobel laureate, 169
    Nobel Prize, 19
    pre-medical school years, 102–4

    refused others' recruiting attempts,
        120–21
    research support from Perot,
        144–45, **152,** 153
    on Seldin's integrity, 67–69
    Smith Kline Beecham, 104
    U.S. National Academy of Sciences
        member, 169
    worked with Dietschy, 111–12
Bryan, John Neely, 20
Buck, Linda, 123
budget
    1910, 31
    1943–1944, xiii
    1949, xiv
    1967, xv, 75
    1985, 125
    2006, xviii
    early 50s, 62
    early 70s, 129
    funding, North Campus building
        project, 159–60
    future challenges, 165–67
    Southwestern Medical Foundation
        assistance, 1951, 71
    Southwestern Medical School, 1951,
        47
    Sprague's building plan, 79
    war years, 45
building. *See also* hospital
    Aston Ambulatory Care Center, xvi
    campus expansion, 1970–1980, xv
    campus expansion, 2000–2006, xvii
    campus, 2006, 7, **161**
    campus, 80s, 128
    (Edward H.) Cary Building for Basic
        Sciences, xiv, 71, **72,** 77
    (Edward H.) Cary Hall, 28–29
    Children's Medical Center, xv, 139
    (Bill and Rita) Clements Advanced
        Medical Imaging Building, xvii,
        160
    (Dan) Danciger Research Building,
        xv, 75, 77
    facilities expansion concept by
        Sprague, 79–80
    Florence Bioinformation Center, xv,
        128

(Tom and Lula) Gooch Auditorium,
 xv, 128
(Cecil H. and Ida) Green Science
 Building, xv, xvi, 128
(Nancy) Hamon Biomedical Re-
 search Building, xvii, 159
(Karl) Hoblitzelle Building for Clini-
 cal Sciences, xiv, 71, **72**, 77
(Philip R.) Jonsson Basic Science Re-
 search Building, xv, 128
land acquisition, xvi
(Eugene) McDermott Academic Ad-
 ministration Building, xv, 128, **129**
Medical Department of the Univer-
 sity of Dallas, **25**
(Harry S.) Moss Clinical Science
 Building, xv, 128
North Campus, xvii, 155, **162**
Ramseur Science Hall, 28, **30**
(Harry) Ransom Center, world-class
 library, 74
(Mary Nell and Ralph B.) Rogers
 Magnetic Resonance Center, 99
(Harold C.) Simmons Biomedical
 Research Building, xvii, 159
(Charles C.) Sprague Clinical Science
 Building, xvi, 98
student facilities, 161–**62**
Burnett, Charles (Chuck), xiv
 departed Southwestern Medical
 School, 48
 recruited Seldin, 53
Burnett, MacFarlin, 84
     C
Cabell, Ben E., 23
Calder, Dr., 21
Caldwell, George, **42**
Campbell Gold Medal, 54
cancer
 Cancer Immunology Center, 87
 chemotherapy, 89–90
 Moncrief Radiation Oncology Build-
  ing, xvii, 159
Capra, Donald, 87
Carnegie
 Corporation, 16
 Foundation for the Advancement of
  Teaching, 14

Institution, 141
Carter, Norman, 107
Cary, Albert Powell, 20
Cary, Edward H., **20, 27, 32**
 Cary Building for Basic Sciences, xiv,
  71, **72, 77**
 Cary Hall, 28–29
 dean, xiii
 dean, Baylor University Medical College, 31
 dean, Southwestern Medical College
  of the Southwestern Medical
  Foundation, 19
 dean, University of Dallas Medical
  Department, 27–28
 early childhood, 20–21
 co-founder, Southwestern Medical
  Foundation, 32–33
 fundraising campaign, early 50s, 36
 medical education, 22–23
 practice in Dallas, 23–24
 University of Texas affiliation,
  46–47
Castle, William, 62
cell biology, 119
 photosynthesis research by Deisenhofer, 132–34
cell biology, department of, xv
 Anderson, chair, 121
 Billingham, chair, 84–85
Chance, Britton, 82
Chapman, Carlton, 107, 148–49
Chapman, John, xi, xii
 affiliation with Baylor University, 28
 contributed to *Principles of Internal
  Medicine*, 43
 on early medical education, 21
 parting from Baylor University, 35
 Southwestern flourishes under Ransom, 74–75
 Southwestern's state of decrepitude,
  early 50s, 55
 Southwestern, 1955, 72
 Sprague as dean, 71, **78**
Children's Medical Center, xv, 139
cholesterol, 110–11. *See also* familial hy-
 percholesterolemia (FH); HMG-CoA
 reductase

cholesterol, *continued*
  research by Siperstein, 65
  statins, 114
Clements (Bill and Rita) Advanced
  Medical Imaging Building, 160, xvii
Clements, Rita, 160
clinical pathology, department of
  Hill, chair, **42**
Cobb, Melanie, 5, xviii
  U.S. National Academy of Sciences
    member, 169
Cold Spring Harbor Laboratory, 130
Columbia University
  Louisa Gross Horwitz Award, 122
Combes, Burton, xii, 67, 107
Cook, Mary McDermott, 153, **154**, 155,
  xii
Cori, Carl and Gerty, 119
Cornell University, 12, 32
Cowan, Maxwell, 6–7
Crick, Francis, 91
Crystal Charity Ball, 147
cyclic AMP, 91–93
  A Protein Binding Assay for Adenosine
    3':5' -Cyclic Monophosphate, 95
  assay, 94–95

D

Dallas. *See also* mayor; Parkland Hospital; philanthropy
  city culture, 45
  civic leaders, founded Southwestern
    Medical Foundation, 33
  Cook, Mary McDermott, 153, **154**
  early medical care in, 20–22
  Hamon, Nancy, **160**
  Jonsson, (John) Erik, 77, **150**
  McDermott, Eugene, 153–55
  O'Donnell, Jr., Peter, 147–51
  perceived as blacklisted after
    Kennedy assassination, 82
  Perot, Ross, 99–101, 144–45, **152**
  philanthropic culture of, 144
  philanthropic leadership, 135
  philanthropists, 1987, 140
  prominent philanthropists and civic
    leaders, **150**
  Rodgers, Woodall, 36
  Rogers, Ralph B., 99–101

Seay, Charles and Sarah, **160**
Simmons, Harold C., 146–47
Southwestern Medical College
  founded in, xiii
Sprague, George, 76
traveling medicine man, Dallas area,
  10
Truett, George W., Pastor, 28
University of Dallas Medical Depart-
  ment, xiii
Dallas County Hospital District, 99
Dallas County Medical Society Alliance's
  Champ Award, 147
Dallas Foundation for Health Education
  and Research, 99
Dallas Medical College, xiii. *See also*
  Baylor University Medical College
Danciger, Dan, 75
  Research Building, xv, 75, **77**
Dealey, Joe M., 80
dean
  Aagaard, George, xiv, **57**
  Alpern, Robert J, xvii
  Bonte, Fred, xv, 87, **88**
  Cary, Edward H., xiii, 31
  Gill, Atticus James (A.J.), xiv, 75–76,
    76
  Gilman, Alfred G., **4**, **90**, 97
  Harrison, Tinsley R., xiv, **43**
  Hart, William Lee, xiv, 57
  Mengert, William F., **44**
  Moursund, Walter, 36
  Moyer, Carl A., xiv, **43**, 57
  Neaves, William B., xvi, 142, **143**
  Rosser, Charles M., **24**, 25–27
  Slaughter, Donald, 41, **42**
  Sprague, Charles C., xv, **78**
  Wildenthal, Kern, xvi, **126**, 127–28
DeGolyer, Everette Lee, 153
Deisenhofer, Johann, xii, xvi, 5
  early education, 132
  Nobel laureate, 169
  photosynthesis research, 132–34
  presentation speech for Nobel Prize
    to, 133–34
  recruited by Sambrook, 133
  U.S. National Academy of Sciences
    member, 169

with wife, Kirsten Fischer-Lindahl,
134
X-ray crystallographer, 132
dermatology, 61
Dietschy, John, 107
cholesterol research, 110
supervised Brown's research, 111–12
Duncan, Charles, 42

E

Earle, Hallie, 26
EDS. *See* Electronic Data Systems (EDS)
Electronic Data Systems (EDS), 152
Eliot, Charles William, 13–14
endocrinology, 53
Endowed Scholar Program, 143–44,
151
enzymology, 92–93
Brown's research, 109–11
HMG-CoA reductase, 111–12, 114
Pfizer Award for Enzyme Chemistry,
122
Siperstein research on HMG-CoA re-
ductase, 111–12
Stadtman, 110
Wieland (Heinrich) Prize for Re-
search in Lipid Metabolism, 122
Estabrook, Ronald W., xii, 80, **81**,
81–83
accomplishments of, 83
dean, Graduate School, 126
Institute of Medicine member, 170
recruited by Sprague, 82–83
U.S. National Academy of Sciences
member, xv, 169
European Molecular Biology Laboratory, 133

F

familial hypercholesterolemia (FH),
110–11, 113. *See also* cholesterol
Goldstein/Brown collaboration on,
115–17
Farmer, Tom, 48, 56
Fashena, Gladys, 43, 45
Federation of American Societies for Ex-
perimental Biology
3M Life Sciences Award, 122
FH. *See* familial hypercholesterolemia
(FH)

Fischer-Lindahl, Kirsten, 133
with husband, Johann Deisenhofer,
134
Flexner, Abraham, xiii, 14, **15**
Florence, Fred F.
co-founder, Southwestern Medical
Foundation, 32–33
Florence Bioinformation Center, xv,
128
Forbes, Gilbert, 44–45
Fordtran, John, xii, 107
on Dallas Medical Department, 26
perception of Seldin's leadership, 67
scholar on early medicine, 23
*Forty Years of Neuroendocrinology: A
Tribute to S.M. McCann,* 80
Foster, Daniel (Dan), **68**, 117, 170
NIH commission, 105
perception of Goldstein, 107
perception of Seldin's leadership, 67
Foundations
Biological Humanics, 155
Carnegie Foundation for the Ad-
vancement of Teaching, 14
Dallas Foundation for Health Educa-
tion and Research, 99
Gladstone, 121
Harold C. Simmons, 146
Hoblitzelle, 36, 38
John D. and Catherine T.
MacArthur, xvi, 157
Johnson Foundation for Medical
Physics, 82
M.D. Anderson, 34
Mayo, 32
McDermott, 140
National Kidney Foundation of
Texas, 147
O'Donnell, 147–48
Parkland, 147
Rockefeller, 16
Shaw Prize, 5
Southwestern Medical, xiii, 32–33,
37, 79, **80**, 128, 149, 155
Susan G. Komen Breast Cancer, 147
Fredrickson, Donald, 115
Friedman, Ben, 43
Fulton, MacDonald, **42**

G

Gairdner Foundation International Award, 97, 122
Gant, Norman F., 170
Garbers, David L., xvii, 169, 170
Gartler, Stanley, 114
gastroenterology, 67, 110
General Education Board, 16
genetic research, 109
  Allan (William) Award, 122
  Brown/Goldstein collaboration on FH, 115–17
  DNA structure, 91
  familial hypercholesterolemia (FH), 110–11, 113, 115–17
  gene cloning, 130
  Seattle Study, 113
Geophysical Research Corporation, 153
Geophysical Services Incorporated (GSI), 153
Gething, Mary Jane, 132
Gill, Atticus James (AJ), xiv, **76**
  dean, UT Southwestern, 75–76
  introduced construction project concept to UT regents, 79
Gilman, Alfred G., xii, xvi, xvii, **90**
  American Academy of Arts and Sciences member, 170
  chair, department of pharmacology, 130
  dean, medical school, xvii
  distinguished awards and honorary degrees, 97
  Institute of Medicine member, 170
  medical education, 91–92
  NIH commission, 105
  Nobel laureate, 169
  Nobel Prize, 3, **4**
  Ph.D. thesis research, 92
  pre-medical school years, 89–91
  Provost, UT Southwestern University, 97, xvii
  recruited to UT Southwestern, 87–89
  U.S. National Academy of Sciences member, 169
Gilman, Kathy, 89
Gilman, Sr., Alfred, 89
Gladstone Foundation, 121

Gladstone, J. David, 121
Goedell, Dave, 142
Goldsmith, Betsy, 133
Goldstein, Joseph L., xii, xv, xvi, 16, 67, **102, 106, 108, 118**
  American Academy of Arts and Sciences member, 170
  awards shared with Brown, 122
  collaboration with Brown, 101, 115–17, 119–20
  genetics research, national reputation in, 113–14
  Institute of Medicine member, 170
  internship and residency with Brown, 108–9
  Journal of Clinical Investigation, 113
  mentored by Siperstein, 65
  NIH research commission, 109–11
  Nobel laureate, 169
  on Seldin's academic clinical medicine, 62
  pre-medical school years, 105–7
  recruited Gilman, 4, 87, 96
  recruited Sambrook, **130–31**
  refused others' recruiting attempts, 119–20
  research support from, 144–45, **152**, 153
  research with Motulsky, 112–14
  U.S. National Academy of Sciences member, 169
Gooch (Tom and Lula) Auditorium, xv, 128
Good Samaritan Hospital, xiii, 25, 29
Goode, John, 55
Goodman and Gilman Award in Drug Receptor Pharmacology, 97
governor, Texas
  Clements, Jr., William P. "Bill," 160
  Neff, Pat Morris, **34**
  Shivers, Robert Allan, 56, **58,** 71
  White, Mark, 148
Grace-New Haven Community Hospital, 51
Green, Cecil, **150**
  establishes Texas Instruments, 153
  philanthropist, 140, 149
  recruited Sprague, 77

Green (Cecil H. and Ida) Science Building, xv, xvi, 128
Green, Ida, **150**
Grollman, Arthur, xiv, 42, **43**
Grundy, Scott M., 170
GSI. *See* Geophysical Services Incorporated (GSI)
Guggenheim Fellowship, 126
Guillemin, Roger, 81
Gustaf, King Carl XVI, **118**

H

Hamilton, C.F., **80**
Hamon, Nancy
    Biomedical Research Building, xvii, 159
    prominent Dallas philanthropist, **160**
Harrison, Betty, 46
Harrison, Tinsley R., xiv, 42–44, **43**
Hart, William Lee, xiv, 57
Harvard Medical School
    exchange program with UT Southwestern residents, 66
Harvard University, 6
    attempt to recruit Brown/Goldstein, 120–21
    attempt to recruit Seldin, 73–75
    Bok, former President Derek, 166
    Civil War era, 12
    Massachusetts General Hospital (MGH), 101–2
    medical school history, 13–14
    Nobel Prize winners, 16
Hazen (Lita Annenberg) Award, 122
Hedland, Kathy, 92
hematology, 77
Hill, Joseph T., **42**
Hindemith, Paul, 53
histology, department of
    Duncan, 42
History of Baylor University College of Medicine, 36
HMG-CoA reductase, 111–12, 114
Hobbs, Helen, 170
Hoblitzelle, Esther, 37
Hoblitzelle, Karl, 37
    Building for Clinical Sciences, xiv, 71, **72,** 77

donated purchase price for medical school land, 36
    Foundation, 33, 37–38, 71
Holmes, Oliver Wendell, 13
hormone research, 91–97
    GTP, 95–96
Horwitz (Louisa Gross) Award, 122
Hospital. *See also* building
    98th General Hospital, 51
    Baylor University Hospital, xiii
    Baylor University Medical Center, 39
    Beth Israel, 73
    first in Dallas, 21
    Good Samaritan Hospital, 25, xiii
    Grace-New Haven Community Hospital, 51
    Massachusetts General (MGH), 101–2
    Parkland, xiii, 17, 18–**19,** 21, 60, 77, **100**
    St. Paul Hospital, 160
    St Paul University Hospital, xvii
    Texas Baptist Memorial Sanitarium, 28
    UT Southwestern University Hospitals, xvii
    Zale Lipshy, 139
    Zale Lipshy University, xvi, **135**
Houston
    Baylor University College of Medicine, 37, 39
    Geophysical Research Corporation, 153
    home of new medical college, 35–36
Howard Hughes Investigators, 6, 131, 133
    McKnight, 141, **142**
Howard Hughes Medical Institute, 133, xvi
    Cowan, 6–7
    UT Southwestern membership, 131
Huber, Robert, 134
Hughes, Howard, 131

I

immunology, 83–85
Indiana University School of Medicine
    Steven C. Beering Award, 97
Institute of Medicine,
    faculty membership list, 170

internal medicine, department of, xiv, xv, xvi, 48
  Burnett, chair, 53
  Chapman, chief of cardiology, 148–49
  Combes, recruited by Seldin, 67
  early 50s, 55
  faculty growth, early Seldin years, 63
  faculty list, 1962, 107
  Foster, chair, **68**
  Harrison, chair, 42, **43**
  at Harvard, offered to Seldin, 73–75
  internationally prominent, 128
  promotional strategies of Seldin, 66
  Seldin, chair, 57
  William Buchanan Chair of, 50
  Wilson, Jean, **64**
  Yale, 49, 53–54
  Ziff, recruited by Seldin, **66**
Intestinal Propulsion in Restrained and Unrestrained Rats, 105
Irvington House Institute for Rheumatic Fever and Allied Diseases, 85

J

John Hopkins University, 6, 32, 108
  Civil War era, 12
  medical school history, 14
Johnson Foundation for Medical Physics, 82
Johnston, John M., 83
Jonsson, (John) Erik, **150**
  cofounder, Texas Instruments, 153
  philanthropist, 140, 149
Jonsson (Philip R.) Basic Science Research Building, xv, 128
Journal of Biological Chemistry, 114
Journal of Clinical Investigation, 113

K

Kaplan, Norman, 107
Karcher, John C., 153
Karolinska Institute, 83
Klein, Jan, 87
Kobler Medal, 50
Komen (Susan G.) Breast Cancer Foundation, 147
Kramer, Robert (Bob), **138**, 139

L

Lasker (Albert) Basic Medical Research Award, 97, 122

Lackey, Robert, **42**
Larner, Joe, 92, 95
Leake, Chauncey, 36
Learning to Heal: The Development of American Medical Education, 9
LeMaistre, Mickey, 158
Lipshy, Ben, 138–39
Lipshy, Bruce, **139**
Lister, George, 170
Lister, Joseph, 10
Looney, William, **42**
Lorenz, Adolf, 29–30
Lounsbery (Richard) Award, 97, 122
Ludmerer, Kenneth, 9
Lynen, Feodor, 114

M

MacArthur (John D. and Catherine T.) Foundation, xvi, 157
MacGregor, George L., 77, **80**
Maddox, Sir John, 122
Marcus, Herbert, 32–33
Mason, Mort, 43
Massachusetts General Hospital (MGH), 101
  group photo of residents, **108**
Max Planck Institute, 132
Mayo Foundation, 32
mayor
  Cabell, Ben E., 23
  Jonsson, J. Erik, 77, **150**
  Rodgers, Woodall, 36
  Sprague, George, 76
McCann, Samuel (Don), 80–81
McConnell, John D., 170
McDermott Foundation, 140
McDermott, Eugene, 77, **80**, 149, **150**
  Academic Administration Building, xv, 128, **129**
  advocacy and support of UT Southwestern, 153–55
  "believed in people," 154
  Center for the Study of Human Growth and Development, 155
  Dallas philanthropist, 153–55
  Endowed chair in anesthesiology, 155
  Foundation, 140
  Plaza and Lecture Rooms, xv
McDermott, Margaret, **154**, 155

McGarry, Dennis, 107
McKnight, Steven L., xii, xvii, **142**
  American Academy of Arts and Sciences member, 170
  businessman and professor, 141–42
  chair, department of biochemistry, 5, 82
  Institute of Medicine member, 170
  recruitment assisted by philanthropic patron, 142–43
  U.S. National Academy of Sciences member, 169
McKusick, Victor, 108
McQuarrie, Irvine, 43–44
Medawar, Sir Peter, 83–84
medical art, department of
  Waters, **42**
Medical Education in the United States and Canada, xiii, 14–16
medical education, U.S. *See also* medical school
  business model of, 166
  Civil War era, **10**–11
  clinical and academic focus, culture class, 13
  during the Civil War, 9–**10**
  Flexner, **15**
  future ethical issues in, 167
  future risks for, 166
  history of, 9–16
  in Dallas, 1800s, 20–22
  rise of the academy and effect on, 12–13
  second-floor letter drops, 21, 24
medical research, U.S. *See also* National Institutes of Health (NIH)
  assisted with funds from NIH, 60
  cancer, 130
  cholesterol metabolism, 65, 110–11, 117–19
  Civil War era, 10–11
  cyclic AMP, 91–93
  European medical training, 12
  hormone, 91–97
  photosynthesis research, 133–34
medical school *See also* dean; medical education, U.S.
  first in Dallas, xiii

Harvard, 13–14, 66
  Southwestern Medical College, xiii
  Stanford University, 5
  Texas College of Physicians and Surgeons, 30
  Stanford University, 5, 120–21
  Tulane University, 76–77
  University of Iowa, 44
  University of Pennsylvania, 101
  University of Washington, 57, 113
  Yale, 49, 52–54
Medical Scientist Training Program (MSTP), **145**–46, 153
Mengert, William F., 44
Michel, Hartmut, 134
Michigan University, 12
microbiology, department of, xiv, xv, xvii, 44
  Fulton, 42
  Sulkin, chair, 44
  Uhr, chair, **85**
Minot, George, 16
Mitchell, Jere, 107
molecular biology, 59–60
  need for leadership in, 130
  V.D. Mattia Award, 122
  X-ray crystallography, 131
molecular biology, department of, xvii
Molecular Cloning: A Laboratory Manual, 130
molecular genetics, department of, xvii, xviii
  Goldstein/Brown collaboration, 121
Moncrief Radiation Oncology Building, xvii, 159
Moncrief, W.A. "Tex," 159
Montgomery III, Philip, 158
Montgomery, Jr., Philip O'Bryan (POB), 58, 148, **148**
Mooney, Booth
  Cary fundraising campaign, 36
  early Cary years, 20
  history, Dallas Medical Department, 26
Moss (Harry S.) Clinical Science Building, xv, 128
Motulsky, Arno, 112–14
Moursund, Walter, 36

Moyer, Carl A., xiv, **43**
    contributed to *Principles of Internal
        Medicine,* 43
    dean, medical school, 57
    professor, experimental surgery, 42
    recruited to Washington University,
        47–48
MSTP. *See* Medical Scientist Training
    Program (MSTP)
Murad, Ferid, 97
Murphy, William, 16
                    N
98th General Hospital, 51
National Heart Institute, 125
National Institutes of Health (NIH), 3
    awarded commission to Brown, 105
    clinical research training for grads, 63
    founded, 60
    Fredrickson, director of, 115
    Medical Scientist Training Program,
        145–46, 153
    Sprague's building plan partially
        funded by, 79
    Wilson, research training at, 65
National Kidney Foundation of Texas,
    147
Neaves, William B., xvi, **143**
    dean, medical school, 3, 142
    North Campus land acquisition, 158
Neff, Pat Morris, **34**
Nestler, Eric J., 170
neurobiology, 91–95
neuroendocrinology
    McCann, Samuel (Don), 80–81
Neurosciences Center, xvii
New York Academy of Sciences
    Award in Biological and Medical Sci-
        ences, 122
New York State Medical Society
    Albion O. Bernstein Award, 122
NIH. *See* National Institutes of Health
    (NIH)
Nirenberg, Marshall, 93–95, 109
Nobel Foundation. *See also* Nobel Prize
    Goldstein/Brown 1985 Award, 117–19
Nobel laureates
    Brown, Michael S., xv, 5
    Burnett, MacFarlin, 84

Deisenhofer, Johann, 5, **134**
Gilman, Alfred, **4, 90,** 97
Goldstein, Joseph L., xv, 5
Medawar, Sir Peter, 83–84
Olson, Eric N., 5
Sudhof, Thomas C., 5
UT Southwestern faculty list of, 169
Nobel Prize, 3–4
    Brown, Michael S., xvi, 99, **102, 118**
    Crick, Francis and Jim Watson, 91
    Deisenhofer, Johann, xvi, 132, **134**
    Gilman, Alfred G., xvii, **4,** 87, **90**
    Goldstein, Joseph L., xvi, 99, **102, 118**
    McCann passed over, 81
    Minot, George, 16
    Murad, Ferid, 97
    Murphy, William, 16
    Nirenberg, Marshall, 94
    presentation speech to Deisenhofer,
        133–34
    presentation speech to Gilman and
        Rodbell, **4,** 96–97
    press release, Brown/Goldstein 1985
        Award, 117–19
    Rodbell, Martin, **4,** 88
    statistics, 5
    Sutherland, Earl W., 97
    Whipple, George, 16
North Campus, xvii, 155
    artist's rendition of future buildings
        on, **162**
    artist's rendition of future hospital
        complex, **163**
    complications with land acquisition,
        158–59
    development sign, **159**
    funding for building project on,
        159–60
    Montgomery helped orchestrate ini-
        tiative, **148**
Northwestern Medical Center, 32
                    O
O'Donnell Foundation, 147–48
O'Donnell, Edith, **147**
O'Donnell, Peter, xii, **147**
    attitude on alumni giving, 149–50
    strong supporter of Texas educa-
        tional system, 147–48

support of UT Southwestern,
148–49
Texan philanthropy, 151
Wildenthal's fundraising style,
150–51
obstetrics and gynecology, department
of
Mengert, chair, **44**
Pritchard, chair, 72, **73**
Olson, Eric N., xvii, 169, 170
On Wings of Eagles, 152
ophthalmology
Cary, Edward Henry, 20–23
Oxford University School of Medicine,
77

P

Parkland Foundation, 147
Parkland Hospital, xiii, xiv, 18–**19, 21,**
55, 77, **100**
during early Seldin years, 60
physical deterioration, 70s, 137–38
state of decrepitude, early 50s, 17,
55–56
Passano Foundation Award, 97, 122
pathology, department of, 148
Caldwell, **42**
Gill, chair, **76**
Montgomery, chair, **148**
pediatrics, department of, 45
penicillin, 49
Pennsylvania State University, 87
Perot, Margot, 152
Perot, Ross, xii, **152**
contribution to strengthen MSTP,
145–46
Dallas civic leader, 99–101
early years, 151–52
Endowed Scholar Program, 151
O'Donnell credits, 149
philanthropist, 140
questions status of UT Health Sciences Center, 122
significant support of medical
school, 144–45
support for UT Southwestern,
140–41
supports "world-class" institutions,
100–101

supports Brown/Goldstein research,
153
Peters, John Punnett, 50–52
Pfizer Award for Enzyme Chemistry,
122
Pharmacological Basis of Therapeutics,
87, 89
pharmacology, department of, xiv, xvi,
xvii, xviii
at University of Virginia, 95
Gilman, chair, **4,** 87–89, **90,** 130
Grollman, chair, 42, **43**
philanthropy
Cary fundraising, early 50s, 36
Cook, Mary McDermott, 153, **154,**
155
Dallas philanthropists, 1987, 140
for medical education, 15–16
generous Dallas civic leadership, 135
Hamon, Nancy, **160**
Hoblitzelle, Karl, 36–**37**
McDermott, Eugene, 77, 80, 149,
150, 153–55
O'Donnell on Texan, 151
Perot, Ross, 99–101, 140–41,
144–46,149, 151, **152–53**
Rogers, Ralph B, 99–101, 149
Seay, Charles and Sarah, 149, **160**
Simmons, Harold and Annette,
146–47
Wildenthal's philosophy on fundrais-
ing, 141
Physiology, Department of, xiv
Grollman, chair, 42, **43**
McCann, chair, 80
Pittman, James, 46
Plass, E.D., 44
porphyria, 61–62
Princeton University Institute for Ad-
vanced Study, 15
*Principles of Internal Medicine (Harri-
son's),* 42–43, xiv
Pritchard, Jack, 72, **73**
*Proceedings of the National Academy of
Sciences,* 95
*Protein Binding Assay for Adenosine 3':5'
-Cyclic Monophosphate,* 95
Prothro, Vin, 158

Public Broadcasting Service, 99
Q
Quantitative Clinical Chemistry, 50
R
rabies, 44
Rall, Edward (Ted), 92, 93
Ramseur Science Hall, 28, **30**
Randall, Joseph, 60
Ransom, Harry Huntt, 73–74
Rector, Fred, 107
Research Institute of Scripps Clinic
    Waterford Award, 97
rheumatology, 109
Rhodopseudomonas viridis, 132
Richard Lounsbery Award, 97, 122
Roche Institute of Molecular Biology
    V.D. Mattia Award, 122
Rochester University, 16
Rockefeller Foundation, 16
Rockefeller Institute, 120–21
Rodbell, Martin, **4**
    awarded Nobel Prize, 3
    hormone research, 95
    Nobel Prize presentation speech,
        96–97
    recruitment attempt of, 88
Rodgers, Woodall, 36
Rogers, Ralph B.
    Dallas civic leader, 99–101
    Magnetic Resonance Center (Mary
        Nell and), 99
    orchestrated bond for new facility,
        138
    Perot's support for UT Southwestern,
        140–41, 152
    philanthropist, 149
Ross, Elliot, 96
Rosser, Charles M., xiii, 23–**24**, 25–**27**
Royal Society of London, xv, 5
    Billingham, Fellow, **84**, 85
    Sambrook, Fellow, **130**
    Russell, David W., xviii, 5, 169
S
Sambrook, Joseph, 5, **130**
    *Molecular Cloning: A Laboratory
        Manual,* 130
    molecular virologist recruited by
        Goldstein, 130–31

recruiting Deisenhofer, 133, **134**
Schally, Andrew, 81
Schein, Lorraine Sulkin, 44
Science, 6
*Scientific Elite: Nobel Laureates in the
    United States, The,* 4
Seattle Study, 113
Seay, Charles, 149
    Dallas civic leader and philanthro-
        pist, **160**
Seay, Sarah
    Dallas civic leader and philanthro-
        pist, **160**
Seay (Charles and Sarah) Biomedical
    Research Building, xvii, 159
Seldin, Donald W., xii, xiv, **18, 50, 51,**
    63
    American Academy of Arts and Sci-
        ences member, 170
    arrival at UT Southwestern Medical
        School, 48
    controversial revision of curriculum,
        61–62
    as entrepreneur, 66
    established metabolic research pro-
        gram, 60
    expert witness in Nazi physician trial,
        52
    "grandfather of UT Southwestern,"
        50
    initial impression of Medical School,
        55
    Institute of Medicine member, 170
    internal faculty recruitment, 62–63
    mentors Goldstein, 107–8
    met Brown, 109
    military service, 51–52
    perception of Sprague, 78–79
    personality of, 62
    philosophy on building Medical
        School, 54–55
    philosophy of clinical scholar, 58–59,
        63–64
    philosophy on recruiting faculty, 53
    pre-medical years, 49
    presidential address, American Soci-
        ety for Clinical Investigation, 59

professorship, Yale Medical School, 52–53
promotional strategies for internal medicine department, 66
recruited Billingham, **84**–85
recruited Combes, 67
recruited Gilman, **4**, 88–89
recruited to UT Southwestern, 53, 54–55
recruiting faculty for UT Southwestern, 57–58
recruitment attempt by Harvard, 73–75
as visionary, 56–57, 59–60
at Yale Medical School, 49–51
Seldin, Muriel, 53, 56
Seymour, Charles, 54
Sharp, Philip, 130
Shaw Prize
Foundation, 5
Wang, Xiaodong, xviii
Shelbourne, Sam, 56
Sheldon, William, 155
Shires, Tom, 137
Shivers, Robert Allan, **58**
political support for building, 56, 71
Simmons, Annette, **146**
numerous awards for civic service, 147
Simmons, Harold C., **146**–47
Biomedical Research Building (Harold C.), 159, xvii
funds for North Campus project, 159
philanthropist, 140, 149
Simmons (Harold C.) Foundation, 146
Simons, Arthur "Bull," 152
Siperstein, Marvin, **65**, 107. *See also* familial hypercholesterolemia
initial contact, Estabrook recruitment, 82
early mentor of Brown and Goldstein, 65
recruiting Billingham, **84**
supervised Brown's research, 111–12
Slaughter, Donald, **42**
dean, Southwestern Medical College, xiii, 41

Small, Andrew, 43
Smith Kline Beecham, 104
Southern Medical Association, 31
Southern Methodist University, 46, 147
Southwestern Medical Association. *See* Cary, Edward H.
Southwestern Medical College of the Southwestern Medical Foundation, xiii, **18**, 19, **38**
financial crisis, mid-40s, 45–46
fulltime faculty and departments, 42
inauspicious beginning of, 34–36
newspaper announcement of accreditation, 35
seal, 35
state of decrepitude, 41, 55, 58
Southwestern Medical Foundation, xiii, 128. *See also* Cary, Edward H.; Hoblitzelle, Karl
Bass, chair, 97
capital improvements fundraising leaders, **80**
charter and founders, 32–33
first location, 37
fundraising with Sprague, 79
O'Donnell credits, 149
role in history of medical school, 155
Southwestern Medical Park Apartments, 161
Southwestern Medical School of the University of Texas, xiv, **25**, **38**
Sulkin, **44**
state of decrepitude, 17–18
statutory branch of the university, 47
Ziff, **66**
Splendid Torch, 99
Sprague, Charles C., xv. **78**, **80**, 127, 149
assisted by Ralph Rogers in fundraising efforts, 99–101
Chair in Medical Science, 98
Clinical Science Building, xvi, 98
Community Service Award, 147
hired Wildenthal as dean, Graduate School, 126–27
pre-medical school, 76
president, UT Health Sciences Center at Dallas, xv, 87

Sprague, Charles C., *continued*
  recruited by Seldin and Dallas civic
    leaders, 77
  recruited faculty, 80–83
  Seldin's opinion of, 78–79
  vision for future facilities expansion,
    79–80
Sprague, George, 76
Sprang, Steve, 133
Srivastava, Deepak, 121
St. Paul Hospital, 160
St. Paul University Hospital, xvii
  future tower complex, **163**
Stadtman, Earl, 110
Stanford University Medical School, 5,
  120–21
Starzl, Tom, 115
Stemmons, John M., 77, **80**
Stevens Institute of Technology, 153
Strauss, Elias, 43
Strauss (Annette G.) Humanitarian
  Award, 147
Streilein, Wayne, 85
Sudhof, Thomas C., xvii, 169
Sulkin, S. Edward, xiv, **44**, 85
surgery, department of, xiv, 55
  Moyer, Carl, 42, **43**
  near collapse of, 137–38
Surgery: Principles and Practice, 48
Sutherland, Jr., Earl W., 91–93, 97
         T
Tamminga, Carol A., 170
Texas. *See also* Dallas; mayor; philan-
  thropy.
  Christian University, 46
  Clements, Jr., Governor William P.
    "Bill", 160
  College of Physicians and Surgeons,
    30
  Dallas' philanthropic culture, 144
  Neff, Governor Pat Morris, **34**
  O'Donnell on Texan philanthropy,
    151
  Shivers, Governor Robert Allan, 56,
    58
  White, Governor Mark, 148
Texas Baptist Memorial Sanitarium, xiii,
  28

Texas Industries, 99
Texas Instruments, 77, 149, 153–54
Thompson, Samuel, 9
Tjian, Robert, 142
Tooze, John, 133
Tower, the, 128
Toxicology Forum, 83
Truett, George W., 28, **29**
Tulane University Medical School, 76
  Dean Charles Sprague, 76–77, **78**
Tularik, 141–42
         U
U.S. National Academy of Sciences, 5–6
  Brown, Michael S., xvi
  Cobb, Melanie, xviii
  Estabrook, Ronald W., xv, 80, **81**, 83
  Garbers, David L., xvii
  Gilman, Alfred G., xvi, **4**, 90, 97
  Goldstein, Joseph L., xvi
  Institute of Medicine, 50, 97, 170
  McKnight, Steven L., xvii, **142**
  Olson, Eric N., xvii
  *Proceedings of the National Academy
    of Sciences*, 95
  Richard Lounsbery Award, 97, 122
  Russell, David W., xviii
  Sudhof, Thomas C., xvii
  Uhr, Jonathan W., xvi, **85**, 87
  Unger, Roger H., xvi
  UT Southwestern faculty member-
    ship list, 169
  Vitetta, Ellen, xvii, 87
  Wilson, Jean D., xvi, 65–66
  Yanagisawa, Masashi, xvii
Uhr, Jonathan W., xii, xv, xvi, **85**, 169,
  170
  first impressions, 86
  recruited by Seldin, 85–86
Unger, Roger H., xvi, 107, 169, 170
*Universities in the Marketplace: The
  Commercialization of Higher Educa-
  tion*, 166
University of California, 121
University of Dallas Medical Depart-
  ment, 25–28
  affiliation with Baylor University,
    28–29
  first medical school in Dallas, xiii

University of Iowa School of Medicine, 44

University of Minnesota Medical School, 44, 57, 71

University of Oklahoma, 87

University of Pennsylvania, 80, 82, 101, 148

University of Texas
  chancellor Ransom, Harry Huntt, 73–74
  chancellor Wilson, Logan, 73
  Committee of Seventy-Five, 72
  Medical Branch, 76

University of Texas Health Sciences Center at Dallas, xv, 122–23, 128

University of Texas MD Anderson Cancer Institute, 158

University of Texas Southwestern Medical Center at Dallas
  name change history, xvi, 18–19
  president, Charles C. Sprague, 78

University of Texas Southwestern Medical School
  Aagaard, 57
  Bonte, 88
  name change to University of Texas Health Science Center at Dallas, 87
  report, UT Committee of Seventy-Five, 72
  research, early Seldin years, 59
  Seldin's controversial revision of curriculum, 61–62

University of Texas Southwestern Medical School: Medical Education in Dallas, 1900–1975, xi

University of the South, 147–48

University of Virginia, 95, 141

University of Washington School of Medicine, 113
  Dean George Aagaard, 57

UT Southwestern. See also Southwestern Medical College of the Southwestern Medical Foundation; Southwestern Medical School of the University of Texas; University of Texas Southwestern Medical School
  academic triumphs, 4–6
  aerial view of campus, 161
  complications, North Campus land acquisition, 158–59
  Dallas civic leadership, 135
  financial position, early 70s, 129
  funding for North Campus building project, 159–60
  future expansion plans, 157–58, 161–62
  future North Campus construction, 162
  future risks in medical research, 165–66
  future St. Paul University Hospital complex, 163
  Estabrook, 83, 81
  Gilman, 4, 87–90, 91–97
  leadership, 1976–1980, 127
  major contributor to, 99–101
  McDermott Center for the Study of Human Growth and Development, 155
  medical school, 6–7, 125
  Medical Scientist Training Program (MSTP), 145–46
  North Campus development sign, 159
  Perot's support for, 140–41, 152
  Rogers' support for, 99–101
  Science, institutional profile, 6
  state of decrepitude, 64, 67
  statistics, current 165
  Wildenthal, 126

UT Southwestern—Commemorating the First Half Century, xi

V

Van Slyke, Donald D., 50

Vitetta, Ellen, xvii, 87, 123, 169, 170

W

Wang, Xiaodong, xviii, 5, 169

Washington and Lee University, 106

Washington University, 77

Waterford Award, 97

Waters, Lewis, 42

Watson, James, 91, 130–31

Weeks, Julius, 127

Weissmann, Gerald, 122

Welch, William H., 12

Western Reserve University, 91, 97
Whipple, George, 16
White, Mark, 148
Wieland (Heinrich) Prize for Research
    in Lipid Metabolism, 122
Wildenthal, Kern, xii, xvi, 3, 149
    asked Seldin to recruit Gilman, 4, 88,
        90
    central administration experience,
        126–27
    challenges to fundraising, 140
    complications, North Campus land
        acquisition, 158–59
    dean, graduate school, 87
    dean, medical center, 126, 128
    desperate need for university hospi-
        tal, 137–38
    early teaching years, 125–26
    fundraising style, 150–51
    Institute of Medicine member, 170
    expansion and McDermotts, 157–58
    philosophy on successful fundraising,
        141, 142–44
    president, xvi, 126
    serious financial crisis, 125
Williams, Dan C., 80
Williams, Paul, 43
Wilson, Jean D., xii, xvi, 64, 107, 170
    advisor to Brown, 116, 117
    appointments of McCann and Es-
        tabrook, 80
    cholesterol absorption, 110–11,
        117–19

faculty departures, 45–46
    inspired by Seldin, 64–65
    NIH research training, 65, 105
    perception of Dallas after Kennedy
        assassination, 82
    perception of Goldstein, 107
    Principles of Internal Medicine (Har-
        rison's), 42–43
    U.S. National Academy of Sciences
        member, 169
Wilson, Logan, 73
        X
X-ray crystallography, 131
        Y
Yale Medical School, 49, 54
    Seldin at, 52–53
Yale Music School, 53
Yale University, 6
    Gilman at, 91
    Seymour, President Charles, 54
Yalow, Rosalyn, 81
Yanagisawa, Masashi, xvii, 5, 169
        Z
Zale Jewelry Company, 138
Zale Lipshy University Hospital, xvi, 99,
        135
    hospital namesakes, 139
    revenue bond financing, 139
Zale, Donald, 138–39
Zale, Morris, 138
Ziff, Morris, 66, 107, 109
Zuckerman, Harriet, 4

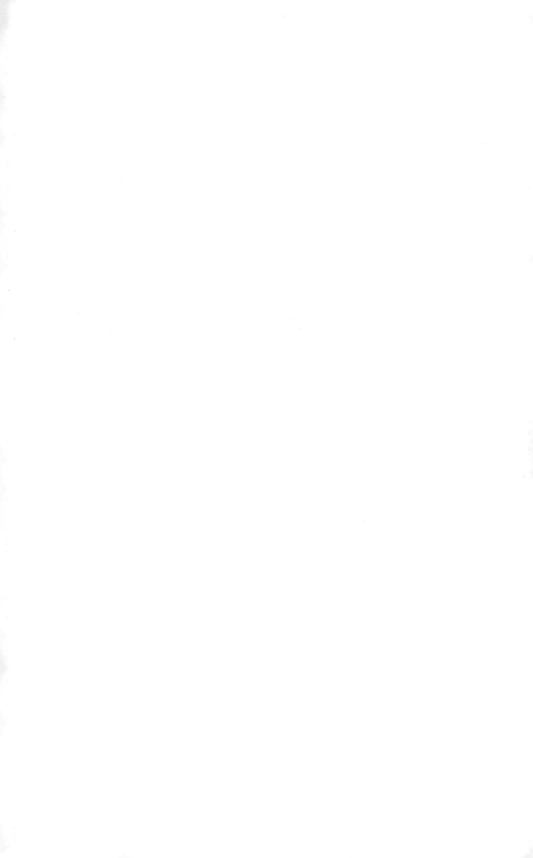